HEAL YOUR CHRONIC PAIN

An Integrated Approach Toward Healing Your Pain

Theven Sabga

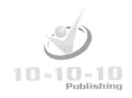

10-10-10
Publishing

HEAL YOUR CHRONIC PAIN: An Integrated Approach Toward Healing Your Pain
www.healyourchronicpain.com
Copyright © 2022 Theven Sabga

Paperback ISBN: 978-1-77277-531-0

Publisher
10-10-10 Publishing

Printed in Canada and the United States of America

This book is dedicated to all
who suffer daily with chronic conditions,
and are ready to break free from the bonds of pain
to seek a life of wellbeing.

I also dedicate this book to my two delightful children,
Talia and Zachary. You are both living examples
of everything this book teaches.

Finally, I dedicate these teachings to the Wisdom teachers
from all traditions, who have disseminated their knowledge
and given us powerful tools to help us achieve
an overall sense of wellbeing in our daily lives.

Table of Contents

Acknowledgements

Many thanks to the following people for their help and inspiration in creating this book:

I want to acknowledge my career as a physiotherapist. The many patients I have worked with who live with chronic pain have taught me so much over the years.

I must thank my husband **Edward**, a medical doctor who has Crohn's disease and faces his own chronic pain issues daily. He teaches me strength and courage. Edward, along with my children, gave me the freedom to write and create this book, with whatever time I needed.

I would like to thank my teachers, especially my yoga teacher, **Yogrishi Vishvketu,** who beautifully brings together an ancient practice for modern times. Thank you to the entire team of coaches at the International Association of Wellness Professionals, for guiding me into approaching health with an integrated approach.

The great folks at Raymond Aaron Publishing: Thank you to **Andreah Barker,** my cherished editor; **Raymond Aaron** himself for making this so seamless; and **Liz Ventrella** for keeping me on track.

On a personal level, many thanks to **Kim Watson,** who guided me through this process; and **Roberto Angelis Lyra** from MuseesuM, who guided me with editing.

Finally, my deepest thanks to my readers, who will continue to surprise me, inspire me, motivate me, and bless me.

Foreword

I s your chronic pain taking control of you? Does it get in the way of your ability to experience joy in your life? Do you feel like there must be a better way to manage your chronic pain?

Are you ready to take control of your life? And step back into the best version of yourself?

If you answered *yes* to any or all of these questions, you have picked up the perfect book. *Heal Your Chronic Pain* gives you the tools you need to become your own pain self-manager.

Theven Sabga has combined years of clinical practice as a physiotherapist with her knowledge of alternative modalities and holistic practices to help you create a well-rounded approach to managing your pain.

No matter where you are in your pain journey, *Heal Your Chronic Pain* is full of insights, and will act as a guide to help you move forward to living and moving more freely. This book flows easily between information sharing and storytelling, making it not only an informative read but an enjoyable one.

Theven shares with you her personal experience so that you can live a happier, healthier and more fulfilling life. Having worked with thousands of patients in her physiotherapy practice, she has witnessed their most common struggles within the healthcare system. Their frustration became hers as well, as she worked to understand why people weren't getting the care they needed. She discovered that, although the system can always work to be better, the true growth needed to happen within the individual.

If you learn to self-manage your own care plan, you are more likely to succeed. Your journey with chronic pain is unique. While many seek to find a quick physical fix, chronic pain is so much more complex. Theven's observations have helped her understand why some are able to get what they need while others get lost in the system. It is all about communication. Being able to communicate what your pain feels like and how it is affecting you physically, spiritually, and emotionally is one of the great gifts you will receive from adopting Theven's approach to pain management.

Heal Your Chronic Pain is about you and for you, the reader who knows your life is about so much more than your pain. Get ready to turn a corner and embark on the next phase of your personal journey. Rewrite your pain story with a happy ending. Theven's compassion, warmth, and breadth of knowledge will be there to guide you every step of the way. The work she inspires will without a doubt change your life. You will walk forward with confidence and strength, knowing you have what you need to live life in JOY!

Raymond Aaron
New York Times **Bestselling Author**

Chapter 1
Achieving a Sense of Hope

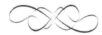

"Pain insists upon being attended to. God whispers to us in our pleasures, speaks in our consciences, but shouts in our pains. It is his megaphone to rouse a deaf world."
– C.S. Lewis

A Brief Overview of Chronic Pain and Self-Management

For over 30 years, in my physiotherapy practice, I have worked with numerous clients living with chronic pain. In the beginning of my practice, I was often left with the feeling that there is so much more to well-being than just physical wellness. In my life, I have faced many of my own challenges. I have learned a lot from my husband, who is a busy emergency room physician, and who also happens to have severe Crohn's disease and yet still manages to remain so positive. I have also learned from my son who survived a benign brain tumor, which caused epilepsy in a young man thriving in the beginning of adulthood. I have learned a lot from myself in the ways I've chosen to deal with my own stress and anxiety. Throughout it all, I have been committed to finding a more balanced approach to living for myself, my family and my patients.

In my work with my clients, I have been inspired by my own journey with yoga, which is a practice that is far from just stretching and exercising the body; yoga is a path to wholeness. Yoga means union of body, mind and soul. I was taught by Himalayan master Yogrishi Vishvketu from Akhanda Yoga, that this holistic approach brings forward an ancient wisdom for a modern age. The practice incorporates asana (positions), pranayama (breathwork), mantra, (sound work), meditation and yogic wisdom in every class. I decided to combine the knowledge learned through yoga with wellness coaching, thus coming up with my holistic approach and signature system: "Heal Your Chronic Pain."

As a physiotherapist, my role is to deal with my patients' physical symptoms, but I could tell that there was so much more I could do to help them end the horrible cycle they were stuck in. It's like a feedback loop that never ends. The good news is, there are ways to help yourself get out of that loop, and not all of them have to do with the physical aspect of the pain. It is now time to consider your emotional, mental, social and spiritual aspects of your pain.

One of the most common complaints I have heard over the years from my patients is that their doctors tell them: "Your pain is all in your head!" This is just poor wording on the part of healthcare professionals (HCPs). It makes the patient feel like they are making it up, or faking it for attention, or being dramatic, or that they are broken in some way. This type of thinking perpetuates a thought loop that can perpetuate and even create disease within the body.

I am sure that when a doctor says, "Your pain is all in your head," it is not meant to be derogatory. They are in a way trying to help their patient see that they don't have to live in pain, but they are unfortunately doing more harm than good with this statement. This way of thinking is so often applied to patients whose injuries do not heal in the expected time frame of current medical models. It is meant in the sense of appreciation that all pain is ultimately in the brain, as the physical cause of the pain has in fact healed.

To help you integrate this understanding, you need to consider the concept of pain as three interacting dimensions:

- Sensory-discriminative
- Cognitive-evaluative
- Motivational-affective

What exactly are these three dimensions?

- The sensory dimension is the awareness of the intensity, location, quality and behaviour of pain.
- The cognitive dimension relates to thoughts about the problem, influenced by experiences and previous knowledge.
- Finally, affective is the emotional response, usually negative, that motivates or governs responses to pain; for example, fear, anxiety, or anger.

All dimensions are essential parts of all pain experiences, and all of these dimensions interact to produce physiological outputs and ultimately altered behaviour.

For example, negative thoughts about an injury and pain arouse negative emotions, which may then arouse neurological and chemical responses potentially impacting on the sensory system. Thus, the negative feedback loop gets reinforced.

Martin, a client I saw with chronic low back pain, was having trouble sleeping at night, which increased his irritability and lowered his motivation during the day. He spent a large portion of his time on the couch watching television. He did not pay much attention to his diet, which also contributed to his overall feeling of low energy. For an energy boost, he would drink 4–6 cups of coffee a day and eat sugary snacks. One day, Martin couldn't take it anymore. He had been fighting the feeling that there had to be more to life for him, and he was ready to stop fighting. He knew life could be better, and he knew he had to be the one to take charge.

During our wellness coaching sessions, we looked at his daily habits, his diet and his before-bedtime routine.

Martin decided that he was drinking too much coffee and switched some of the cups he was drinking to decaffeinated, which over time he replaced with herbal teas. By drinking coffee all day, he was dehydrated at night and was drinking too much water before bed, which caused frequent waking to use the bathroom. He reduced his television intake before bed and replaced it with reading and then breathwork techniques. He then adjusted the temperature of his house before bed, because he realized that in order to sleep, he needed to have a cool room.

By improving his quality of sleep, he found that he had more energy during the day, and he developed a routine of slow stretches. By paying attention to his diet, he was able to opt for more nourishing whole foods rather than processed food .

Martin identified that this did not take willpower to change; it was the realization of how he was contributing to the vicious cycle, and it was his willingness to change this pattern that allowed him to make the lifestyle changes that were more life enhancing for him.

A good attitude cannot cure your chronic pain; however, a positive attitude and certain self-management skills can make it much easier to live with.

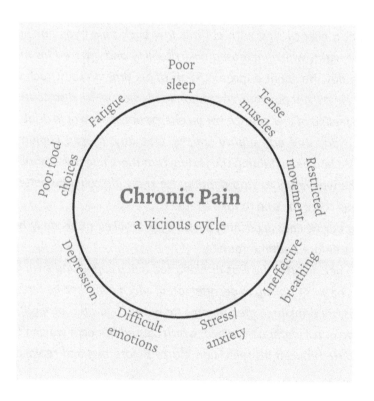

You Have the Power to Choose

"Your life is yours to live, no matter how you choose to live it.
When you do not think about how you intend to live it, it lives you.
When you occupy it, step into it consciously, you live it."
– Gary Zukav

I believe you picked up this book because you are ready to choose a life beyond pain. You are ready to stop allowing your pain to control your life and steal away your joy. You are ready to take your power back.

Nobody wants to live with chronic pain. But unfortunately, many do. Some types of chronic pain have easily identifiable sources, and some don't. I wrote this book with a holistic approach in mind. I have witnessed and believe without a shadow of a doubt that there are healthy ways to manage your pain, and that you can in fact enjoy a more fulfilling and satisfying life. This may seem contradictory to you, especially if you have been living with chronic pain for years now.

You may ask, "How can I live a healthier, happier life when I am in pain?" Whether you are dealing with the challenges of chronic conditions like low back pain, fibromyalgia, heart disease, or depression, you can choose an approach that helps you alleviate your anxiety, achieve better sleep patterns, and regain your strength. But most importantly, when you give yourself the right tools and take control of your pain, you ultimately allow yourself to feel hope again.

A healthy way to live with chronic pain is to work at managing the physical, mental, and emotional dimensions caused by the condition. With identifying your challenges, you can then problem solve and set goals. Your goals need to be tangible and achievable. Your goals will be personal to you. Sometimes they will be big and sometimes they will be small, like getting out of bed in the morning and getting dressed. As you read this book and continue to understand that you are in control, no matter how hard that might be to believe right now, release all judgement of yourself. You are always doing the best you can with what you have in the moment. I am here to help you learn more so that you can do more. So, if you got out of bed today, when you would've rather pulled the blankets back over your head, I congratulate you. You did it! Keep going.

This book is intended to provide you with information on the multidimensional causes of pain, and to enable you to use your power of awareness. When you are done, you will understand the things you can control. You will be able to control those things because you will have equipped yourself with positive coping skills.

Most human beings do not realize the tremendous power of two incredible gifts they have been given on this Earth:

1. The power to self-heal
2. Creativity

You have the power to heal yourself. You are a creative being who can use this skill to help you not only find solutions that work for you, but to take your life experience and creatively reimagine it. You have the ability to write your next chapter, and that chapter can be the best of your life if you choose it to be.

When you believe you are limited, then anything you envision or create will be limited, but if you can see that your ability to respond is limitless, your internal power is enhanced. You have the opportunity in this very moment to transcend your limitations of thought, emotion, and action, and consciously craft yourself to become the creation you want to be.

Pain Is a Multi-Dimensional Experience

There is no one "pain centre" in the brain. There are billions of nerve cells in the spinal cord and in many areas of the brain that are involved with pain. It is important for and your family to understand the differences between acute and chronic pain because an informed system is an important part of successful self-management of pain.

What is acute pain?

1. Acute pain has an identifiable cause.
2. It is usually only felt for a short period of time, within the frame of the body's healing mechanism. We have all experienced acute pain at some point: a cut finger, a sore throat, or a sprained ankle are just a few examples.
3. The pain occurs in a specific area of the body.
4. It usually goes away once healing has taken place.
5. Acute pain has survival goals. It's our body's efficient way of warning us of danger and harm. The body usually reacts to protect. If something hurts, we stop and rest and allow healing to take place. As the pain subsides and healing takes place, the body's protective mechanisms decrease.
6. With acute pain, you gradually increase your activity and return back to normal within the time frame of healing.

When Acute Pain Becomes Chronic

In some cases, the pain symptoms caused by acute pain do not diminish even though the physical healing has occurred. The brain network continues to interpret the nerve impulses as "dangerous," and a feedback loop is initiated. I will explain more about this feedback loop and how you can interrupt or manage it, throughout this book.

What is chronic pain?

Chronic pain is defined as pain lasting longer than six months, which is longer than the normal time frame for healing and recovery.

There are two types of chronic pain:

1. The first type is associated with chronic disease; for example, osteo-arthritis, rheumatoid arthritis, or gout, etc. The medical management for this type of pain is specific to the disease, as this type of chronic pain happens when chronically weakened tissue is mechanically threatened. Thus, health and protection of the tissues is necessary. That said, there are still a whole myriad of holistic approaches that I will share, which will also help you take control of this type of pain.

2. The second cause of chronic pain is called idiopathic, meaning there is no known cause for the pain. Some examples of idiopathic pain are persistent headaches, chronic neck pain, shoulder pain, lower back pain, fibro-myalgia, and chronic pelvic pain. This type of pain can range from mild to severe and can be felt in one or many areas of the body.

Your Brain Has the Power to Heal

At the beginning of this chapter, I talked about how so many clients I have worked with have been frustrated by their doctors telling them that their pain is all in their head. I understand why that would be frustrating. Yes, your brain triggers a pain response in your body, sometimes based off of inaccurate information; however, the pain that is felt throughout the body is very real, which means that the pain is not just in your head, because you are feeling it. Chronic pain causes never-ending stress. It causes ongoing irritability, fatigue, isolation, and an overall feeling of helplessness. When a doctor tells you it's all in your head but doesn't give you the tools to change your negative pain-causing thought loops, that pain continues to exist in your body.

When dealing with chronic pain, I have learned that there are many approaches that can be used to disrupt that pattern. Your over-arching goal is to soothe the nervous system and retrain the brain. The work you will begin to do in this is the beginning of your inner reprogramming. This is not a term that I've created myself; I've actually learned it from my own yoga teacher and have found it to be incredibly powerful in my own life.

The good news is that you can do many things to calm the nervous system and work on your inner reprogramming. The brain is like your own personal pharmacy. When you need some medicine in daily life, you go in and ask for it. The same thing needs to happen in your brain. When you need some medicine to heal, you need to trigger your brain to release the neurochemicals you require to heal. This can be done through understanding your disease process. When you understand what needs to be healed, you'll begin to learn how best to heal it. You'll begin to create a self-healing practice that works best for you personally, one that will involve things like self-pacing, mindful exercise, relaxation and meditation, yoga, eating for nourishment, and getting the support you need.

The Science of Pain

As you probably already know, nerves in our body are like electrical wires that signal the brain. The nerves are the things that let your brain know when a certain stimulus is harmful. Let's say you cut your finger. Within seconds of the knife grazing your skin, the nerve endings send an impulse to the spinal cord. Your spinal cord is like the superhighway of information, connecting your nerves to your brain.

Your brain receives the signal and then asks the question: "Is this dangerous?" If the nerves reply that it is, the brain sends out a warning and you feel the pain. YES, the pain is interpreted by your brain to signal the body into action; therefore, all pain is experienced in the brain.

In Melzack and Wall's *Gate Control Theory,* they describe a transmission station in the spinal cord that is likened to a gate. Two things can happen when pain is transmitted:

1. If the gate is open, the impulses pass through and continue up the spinal cord to the brain. If the brain senses danger from the impulses, you experience pain.

2. If the gate is closed or even partially closed, then only some or none of the impulses travel to the brain. The brain might interpret this as little or no danger, so you experience minimal or no pain.

The gates of your spinal information highway can be opened or closed in many ways, and the brain plays a huge role. The brain can send nerve impulses to close or open the gate. Some of the key factors that influence your brain's decision-making process are:

- Past experience.
- Feelings surrounding pain.
- Beliefs about pain.
- Expectations about what will happen.
- The amount of attention we give to the pain.
- Emotions.

The pain gates can be closed by things like a resilient and positive mindset, using distraction, and deep abdominal breathing, which will reduce the perception of fear; while the pain gates can be held open by anxiety and fear, which serves to amplify the pain.

I hope you are beginning to understand that pain is multidimensional and that your interpretation of pain comes from information exchanges within your entire nervous system. Most of these areas are within our control. When you bring awareness to how you are reacting to your emotions, thoughts, and the processing of your body's sensations—being touched, seeing, hearing, tasting, and smelling—you give yourself the ability to begin to truly understand your pain. You begin to see the pattern of nerve impulses created by how you experience pain, the action your body takes to protect you from perceived danger, and how the neurochemicals released from your brain can help regulate the stress caused by pain.

One of the most important take-aways from this chapter is the knowledge that pain is either caused, increased, or decreased by its assessment of the danger you are in. It is not always the result of an injury.

Science supports the important role of our thoughts, emotions, and physical sensations in the role of our perception of pain. Throughout this book, I will lean into the science to explain how a positive mindset, mindful movement, deep breathing, healthy eating, and many other factors can help close the gate to habitual patterns of perceived danger and therefore greater pain.

Break the Cycle of Chronic Pain

Chronic pain is a disturbance. It is a disturbance of your complex interactive neurological system. It is a disturbance of your immune system. It is a disturbance of your stress response system. It is a disturbance of your genetic makeup. It is a disturbance of your life. When chronic pain continues to last in your body, the pain has no survival value. If the ongoing pain is not managed, it might be causing a reduction in the quality of life. You can choose to lie in bed and take medications; that is certainly one way of management. Or you can bring understanding and a greater awareness to the process and equip yourself to be a positive self-manager of these symptoms.

13

What are the symptoms of chronic pain?

Knowing what you are feeling and why you are feeling these things is an important first step in becoming a positive self-manager. It is here that you will begin to break the vicious cycle of chronic pain.

Chronic pain is generally accompanied by a whole host of differing symptoms. You may feel that your pain alone is causing you to feel tired and fatigued, to have restricted motion due to joint and muscle pain, and to feel in a low mood. It's important to note that these symptoms can feed off of each other. For example, fear and anxiety about the future with this ongoing pain can result in you tensing your muscles, leading to lack of movement, poor sleep, fatigue, and poor eating habits. Feeling this bad can cause you to withdraw from your friends, your family, and your life.

Same Chronic Conditions, Different Perspectives

Let's take a brief moment to talk about perspective. We've all experienced how a change in perspective can shift any situation. If you left a conversation being angry with someone you love, and allow yourself to reflect on what happened, you can often see where they are coming from even if you still don't agree with them. That shift in perspective may allow you to have a more meaningful conversation with them about what made you angry. The same is true of your chronic pain. Shift your perspective, and I promise you will see an improvement in your quality of life.

Here are two quick examples of clients I have worked with, to help you see what I mean here:

Phyllis, 48, had a hip replacement and also suffers from chronic low back pain. She has retired from work and spends most of her time sleeping or watching television. She is scared of physical activity because she is worried it will cause more harm. She has problems sleeping at night, feels fatigued, and

14

mostly eats fast and processed foods. Phyllis has developed social anxiety. She feels like a burden to her family and thinks that they would rather not be around her. Phyllis has allowed her chronic pain to drastically lower her quality of life.

Carol, 58, suffers from chronic hip pain caused by a failed hip surgery, and chronic low back pain. During the summer months, she swims, follows a customized exercise routine, and does chair yoga. She has learned to listen to her body and understands that pacing her activities around doing what she enjoys is key, so she can still do what she loves. She has a very curious mind and questions new symptoms as they arise. Rather than dwelling on the new problem, she finds a way to solve it. Because she had taken control of her pain, Carol still enjoys all that life has to offer her, including going camping with her husband.

The big difference between the two examples I just shared was that one of my clients decided to embrace adversity. There are plenty of times in life when we all face adversity. Each tough time you face, the universe is asking you to learn a lesson. The harder the lesson, the harder it might be to get through. Even if you feel that your world is falling apart, don't give up! Look at the situation as something you have to rise above and resolve to come out of it on a positive note. You gain a sense of strength in yourself by embracing adversity. You may not feel this while you are in the middle of a situation, but you are becoming a stronger person because of what you are going through.

Embracing adversity isn't easy by any means, but it will allow you to see different possibilities within your life and to examine your reactions to situations. Adversity is a teacher. You may not always like the teacher, but it does not change the fact that there is a lesson to be learned. Adversity often shows its face right before you're about to make a major breakthrough.

The time is now. Look at the challenges you are facing today as soul strengthening.

10 Points to Be Aware of as You Heal Your Chronic Pain

1. YOU ARE NOT ALONE!

You may be feeling that your pain is invisible—because people can't see it, they don't believe it is real. I know it is real. I also know that there are many in the same situation as you. Therefore, surrounding yourself with like-minded people, who are going through the same thing, can reduce the feeling of isolation. Reaching out can give you the opportunity to help others, as well as recognize your own resilience and coping skills, and in turn can help you with strategies and tips.

It's important to not do this alone, and finding this support can come from reading a book as you are doing now, reaching out to a healthcare professional, or attending support groups, of which there are many online now as well.

2. YOU ARE NOT RESPONSIBLE FOR CREATING YOUR CHRONIC PAIN

Understand that your pain is multidimensional and caused by many factors. Having an understanding now of the mechanisms of how pain manifests itself can help you become a better self-manager. You are beginning to learn how to work with your pain rather than against it.

3. DON'T GET CAUGHT UP IN YOUR THOUGHTS

It's so easy to become involved in your thoughts. You think that your thoughts are your fundamental nature. You overidentify with your thoughts and lose touch with that deeper sense of being, that deeper witness consciousness. Give your thoughts recognition, but practice becoming curious about them. Observe your thoughts; don't live in them. Instead of riding the wave of thoughts and reacting, try becoming introspective. Slow down and come back to the breath; notice the space between the thoughts, and fall back

16

into the present moment. Then with kindness to yourself, make a conscious choice to respond using the tools you know now and will come to know.

4. STILLNESS COMES WITH PRACTICE

Learning to unwind the thoughts and habitual patterns comes only with practice. In yogic tradition, this practice is called abhyasa, and the un-entanglement with thoughts is vairagya.

Abhyasa is defined as the slight effort to remain present, noticing the air on the skin, noticing sound and smell and textures around you, and coming back to the breath. Un-entanglement (vairagya) is the art of surrendering and letting go. This does not mean a disinterest, or that you withdraw, or that you turn your back on life, which in a way denies the difficulty of life. To unentangle means that you can stand in the middle of chaos and confusion and noise and remain present to what is and to yourself.

5. MEMORIES ARE A COLLECTION OF PAST EXPERIENCES

Memory can be the source of ongoing context for all of our future experiences. Memories can inform and positively or negatively affect our future actions. When you live in the past, you may have regret or fear, and so when you overthink the future, you are wrought with worry. Practice being in the present moment. Being fully engaged gives you the power to change.

6. YOU ARE NOT YOUR PAIN

Are you aware that you are more than this body-mind complex? You are essentially pure awareness and consciousness. Ask yourself these questions:

1. Are you aware of your body, or is your body aware of you?
2. Are you aware of your thoughts, or are your thoughts aware of you?

What do these questions mean? Your awareness belongs to you; you are the subject. Your body and mind are objects to that subject. You are the awareness functioning through this body-mind complex. You are pure awareness. Thought is yours, but it's not you. Use the body and mind as a tool to your purpose. There is an abundance of power and wisdom available to you through your awareness and consciousness. All you have to do is notice it and relax into it.

7. MANAGE YOURSELF, MANAGE YOUR LIFE

Self-management is a choice. You can either choose to become an active self-manager or do nothing and suffer in silence. It's important to have a mission in life. Most people realize their purpose through adversity. It is not the only way to realize one's purpose but probably one of the most common routes.

Ask yourself the following questions to help you set your intention with your healing practice going forward:

* How would I like today to unfold?
* What would I like to focus my energy and attention on?
* What brings me joy?
* What makes me feel balanced?
* What state of mind would I like to be in?

Get curious about your answers. Setting an intention to your practice is the momentum and energy you need to help you achieve your goals.

8. TAKE TIME FOR REFLECTION

Connect to your inner wisdom and let that be your guide. The brain is neuroplastic and can be remolded by practicing and changing habitual patterns. When you slow down to reflect, you can settle the mind and drop into the spacious awareness that underlies the routine of day-to-day functioning.

9. CONTINUOUS CARE AND ATTENTION, OVER TIME, ESTABLISHES YOUR PRACTICE

Having a strong intention is what fuels you and gives you the momentum to move forward. Caring for yourself and paying attention to your situation, moment by moment, grounds you in awareness. Your bodily systems work through rhythm and repetition. Focusing on regular patterns, like intentional breathing, brings a sense of balance, whereas irregular patterns, like jagged and heavy breathing, can bring anxiety. To come back to a place of calm, notice your breath. Commit to using this tool when thoughts are running away. As we work through the remaining chapters of this book, I will provide more tools for quieting your mind and, over time, you will begin to find it easier.

10. DEVELOP COMPASSION FOR YOURSELF AND OTHERS

Some people worry that self-compassion will make them soft, but it actually gives us incredible power. Be your own best friend; be there for yourself. Treat your pain or low mood with curiosity and gentleness. When you are mindful of your path, you show up for your pain, and you honour its presence. You will find ways to just be with it. Healing is about self-empowerment. You have all the tools within you. Self-compassion isn't about pushing through or ignoring difficult emotions; it means encountering these feelings—not to control them but to change your relationship to them. Moments of self-compassion are accompanied by feelings of ease, comfort, and encouragement.

- Be your own best friend.

- Be your own advocate.
- Be your own biggest fan.
- Love yourself more than anyone else in the world.
- Give yourself the tools to heal.
- Become your own self-manager and take control of your life!

Chapter 2
Your Wellness Wheel

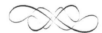

*"For everyone, well-being is a journey.
The secret is committing to that journey and taking
those first steps with hope and belief in yourself."*
– Deepak Chopra

Have you gone through a time in your life when everything feels out of balance? You feel like you are doing so much, and your efforts are not producing the gains you want? There is so much to be done and no time to do it. It doesn't matter how hard you work in the day; you consistently feel like you can't do enough. You feel exhausted. You feel like your body is breaking down. Maybe you are going through this right now, and this is why you've reached for this book.

I'm glad you are here. I personally have gone through a time like that in my own life, and it gave me even more inspiration to find a method of understanding to what wellness really means. What does true wellness mean to you? What does total health feel like to you?

In this chapter, I am going to share with you the principal that governs my approach to Wellness Coaching: The Triangle of Health. I will then tie this concept to the layers of the Wellness 360 Wheel.

Within my own wellness coaching journey, I have found a way to deal with the challenges I face in my own life. My journey to developing the work I do, to achieve holistic wellness in all areas of my life, has helped me to more effectively manage my stress, overwhelm, and weight gain. I have learned how to manage my time so that I have more for myself. I have also discovered how to live my life with purpose and passion. When I hear that inner critic trying to rear its ugly head, I now have the tools to access that powerful inner creator.

I know I am not alone when I tell you that there have been times in my life when that inner critic, the overwhelm, the stress, the anxiety, have all gotten to me. The difference now is that I have given myself the strength, knowledge, and power to deal with these moments in healthy ways. I am sharing a philosophy with you that shifted my life in profound ways.

The most transformative thing you can do for yourself, and your life, is to do something you love. Find your passion and your purpose. This is the foundation for everything. When you wake up in the morning excited to do the work you do, it inspires you to feel better. In my experience, I have found that when you do something you love that fills you with purpose, you will be happier and more successful doing it. When your willpower is struggling, having an intention toward why you are doing it can really empower your willingness to achieve it when the going gets tough.

Think of this chapter like a workbook. The goal for you is to discover what layers of your life are out of balance, so that you have a clear starting place for your work going forward. You have to know your starting place in order to map your course. This is where you are now. At the beginning. In the discovery stage. Your goal in this work is to be honest with yourself. Own where you are at, so that you can move forward to a place of holistic wellness.

What Is Wellness Coaching?

Essentially, as a wellness coach, I help you understand what your own wellness means to you and how to achieve total health. The work I do helps you build a strong foundation through understanding the different elements that make up your wellness. This is a revolutionary approach to life. This is a philosophy, not a prescription.

So how do you solve a health challenge? A system (meaning something that is not personalized) or a Band-Aid solution usually only addresses part of the problem. When it comes to wellness, rigid systems do not work. They might work for a while, but they do not take into account the whole picture. You are ever-changing, and you need a unique program that is flexible and based on a true holistic view of your life. Wellness coaching provides you with a holistic system that works for the long term, because it does both of those things, allowing you to evolve. You are given a roadmap, and there may be more than one path to follow, but you are the driver.

Wellness coaching takes a 360 view of all the elements of your health. There is no cookie-cutter solution to you, as you are ever-changing; thus, it is very revealing to apply a wellness 360 approach to your health. At first glance, when you look at the 12 elements of wellness on the 360 wheel, it is important to note that these elements are not viewed in isolation but rather all together, as the elements interact with each other. This is a true holistic perspective that gives you a deeper understanding of yourself, so that you can make a lasting change and transformation. This approach is dynamic, not static. We can all live in extreme imbalance; however, we can use the wellness 360 perspective to bring us back into balance.

Finding balance is an elusive statement. We can find it for short periods of time, but we need to have the right tools in our toolbox to bring us back. This process needs constant refinement.

The Wellness 360 Wheel

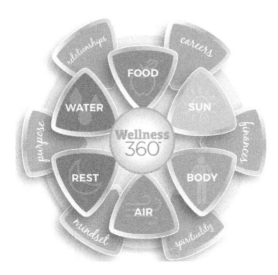

Wellness coaching takes a 360 view of your complete health and wellness. It considers every aspect of your life. I believe all of these require attention in order to create more well-being. This includes your nutrition and exercise, as well as your relationships, career, quality of sleep, and so much more. If one element is out of balance, they all are, so taking a broad view allows you to get to the core of the issues you are facing in order to overcome them.

The Triangle of Health

"Through the vehicle of our emotions, our mind, body, and spirit are sending signals that something has to shift."
– Deepak Chopra

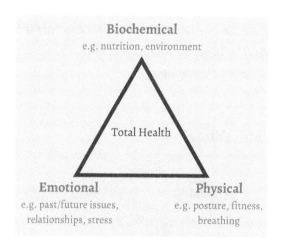

Your health and well-being are governed by three elements in constant flux:

"On the first layer—**the physical, external layer**—Wellness 360 continues to provide a holistic framework for balancing our lives in the 12 elements of life we originally created.

On the second layer—**the internal, inner layer**—Wellness 360 goes to the next level by integrating both the external and internal. We are not just physical bodies; we have an internal world that plays a huge role in our health. What's happening on the inside is often as important as what is happening on the outside.

And finally, on the third layer—**the symbolic, more "energetic"** layer or that hidden layer you can't see—Wellness 360 provides greater meaning to the areas of our lives that are out of balance, and provides a deeper understanding of our individual journeys."[1]

Together, they form the three corners of a triangle, which represents your total health. As you work through the questions in this chapter, keep in mind that what total health means is unique. The basic definition of wellness is:

"The state of being in good health, especially as an actively pursued goal."

But what that means for you will look very different from what it looks like for me or for your neighbour or your partner or even your children. For some, it means being able to hike mountains, while for others it means being able to play with their children. For some, it means writing books, while for others it means being able to sit in quiet contemplation. The life you live as the healthiest version of you is deeply personal. Embrace who you are. Embrace your needs. Listen to your body. Listen to your soul. Listen to that little feeling in the pit of your stomach that tells you to go for it. Get excited!

Wellness 360 and the Triangle of Health

This triangle governs my wellness coaching approach to healing. I use the triangle to then dive more into the elements on the Wellness Wheel. With each element on the Wellness Wheel, we take a three-dimensional perspective that supports you as a whole.

---

1 https://iawpwellnesscoach.com

Using the Wellness 360 Wheel, combined with the triangle of health, you can figure out the root cause of the problems you are facing right now. Let's focus on the 12 elements of the Wellness 360 Wheel for a moment, which are food, sun, body, air, rest, water, relationships, careers, finances, spirituality, mindset, and purpose. All of the elements on the 360 Wheel are interconnected. Each element interacts with the others, which contributes to our well-being as a whole. Wellness coaching takes a holistic view of all these elements to achieve true balance.

Wellness 360 is a philosophy that I learned as a wellness coach, from the International Association of Wellness Professionals (IAWP)[2]. Its basic principle is that our health and well-being is affected by all areas of our lives. Beyond our nutrition, there are many other factors that affect our overall wellness. We can't just look at health in a vacuum; rather, we need to look at the whole picture.

Having a 360-degree perspective when you look at yourself will help you to see how one area of your life may be affecting another area. This interconnection between all parts of ourselves is truly a holistic approach to wellness. Wellness 360 reminds us that we are whole beings with a variety of influences upon our being. We are also not just physical beings; we have multiple facets to ourselves. When we change one area of our lives, we often see other areas change. When we struggle in one area, we often see a direct impact upon another area. Knowing how everything is connected, we can better prepare ourselves for creating more balance and lasting changes. Wellness 360 also points to the fact that we are all unique and have unique needs.

The inner wheel represents elements that affect your health directly: food, sun, body, air, rest, and water. For example, if you aren't providing your body with enough nutrients with the food you eat, your health will eventually come out of balance. The same is true if you are not breathing in good air or getting enough rest. If you are not paying attention to the needs of your body, you

2 https://internationalassociationofwellnessprofessionals.org

will inevitably create an imbalance that needs to be corrected.

The outer wheel consists of six elements: careers, finances, spirituality, mindset, purpose, and relationships. These elements are the indirect elements that affect a person's health and well-being. They are considered to be indirect because they are not always the first thing a person considers when wanting to achieve a healthy lifestyle.

Both the inner wheel and the outer wheel play significant roles in creating a truly healthy, holistic lifestyle. As you do the work, continue to keep in mind that all of the elements of the wheel do not act alone. Often, one element of the wheel impacts another. The Wellness 360 Wheel helps us to understand how the elements of our lives are interconnected and how we can approach our lives holistically to create lasting changes. These changes are ones that impact our overall lives rather than acting as quick fixes that can be achieved by only looking at one element in isolation.

The multi-layered perspective of Wellness 360 expands the understanding of each element beyond the basic, physical level. We continue to work with the whole triangle and also explore each element on a mental and emotional level. This is holistic health.

Holistic health is an approach quite different from mainstream medicine, which takes an allopathic perspective to treating an illness. Allopathic approaches attempt to fight, reduce, or suppress either the disease itself or isolated symptoms of the disease, through the use of drugs or surgical methods. Often, it follows a strict biochemical definition of food and nutrition alone.

Holism instead looks at the entire state of the body as the bigger picture and seeks to strengthen its own ability to fight disease on its own, more so with natural methods. This extends to spiritual, emotional, and other states of health for the greatest impact.

Wellness Score

This exercise has been taken from my studies with IAWP. It is one that I use regularly with my clients and have found to be very effective.

Give yourself 1 point for each of the following statements that are true to your own personal behaviours. If the statement is not true, give yourself a 0.

- *I eat more fresh, whole foods than processed foods.*
- *I engage in some type of physical activity each day.*
- *I experience a restful sleep most of the time.*
- *I spend some time outside each day.*
- *I do not smoke nor breathe in second-hand smoke.*
- *I drink 6 glasses of water per day.*
- *I feel good about the personal relationships I have.*
- *I enjoy my career.*
- *I feel financially secure.*
- *I am not stressed out.*
- *I have a spiritual practice that is a part of my life.*
- *I feel I have a purpose in life.*

Total the number of points from the quiz above and read the scoring below to better understand your score.

If you scored 10

Congratulations! Your current Wellness Score is fairly balanced. You are likely someone who is eating well, exercising, and is focused on improving other areas of your life that affect your well-being. If some areas may still be out of balance, use the Wellness 360 Wheel below to determine which areas still need support.

If you scored between 6 and 9

You're on your way. You have some strong foundations in place for your health, but you are still working to improve other areas. Identifying which areas need further support will greatly benefit you. Choose one area at a time to focus on improving by using the Wellness 360 Wheel below.

If you scored less than 6

Time to set priorities. While you may feel that some areas of your health are going okay, there are areas that need some attention. Don't tackle them all at once, but rather choose one area at a time to focus on. Consider getting support from a trained professional or wellness coach in the areas you would like to improve.

Wellness 360 is the IAWP philosophy that our health and well-being is affected by all areas of our lives. Beyond the food we eat, there are many other factors that affect our overall wellness. We can't just look at health in a vacuum, but rather we need to look at the whole picture. Wellness 360 takes into account all areas of a person's life that directly impact one's health, including physical factors such as sunshine, air, sleep, movement, food, and water, and non-physical elements, including relationships, career, finances, mindset, spirituality, and purpose.

Having a 360-degree perspective when you look at yourself will help you to see how one area of your life may be affecting another area. This inter-connection between all parts of ourselves is truly a holistic approach to wellness. Wellness 360 reminds us that we are whole beings with a variety of influences upon our being. When we change one area of our lives, we often see other areas change. When we struggle in one area, we often seen a direct impact upon another area. Knowing how everything is connected, we can better prepare ourselves for creating more balance and lasting changes. Wellness 360 also points to the fact that we are all unique and have unique needs. What works for one person may not work for another, simply because one element of their life is different. The good news is, we don't have to do advanced medical testing to figure out why they are different. We can simply take the Wellness 360-degree approach to find out what is in balance and what is out of balance, and work to make small changes to reach our goals.[3]

Your Physical State

You know that your physical health is about so much more than just your physical state of being. In the first chapter, I talked a lot about how our brain can affect the experience of chronic pain. The physical sensation is real. The physically feeling of pain is life-altering. Pain affects the whole triangle. When you are living with chronic pain, it affects you mentally and emotionally as well. How you feel about yourself, how you walk into the world, and the choices you make are all affected by the pain.

Each of the 12 areas of the Wellness 360 Wheel affect your physical state. The most important ones to connect are the ones on the inner wheel. When you take time to walk in the sun, you physically feel better because it helps your immune system to fight disease. When you drink enough water, you are helping your body achieve optimal health. When you listen to the needs of your body, you are making your physical health a priority.

Daily Body Scan – This is where you can begin with the element of body to start connecting to the messages your body is sending you.

You are going to continue your work in this chapter by doing something called a body scan. This is an exercise that I've taken from my learning with IAWP. It only takes a few minutes and it's best to do it every day. Don't overthink it; just close your eyes and listen to your body.

---

[3] https://iawpwellnesscoach.com/wellness-coaching/

Instructions:

1. Find a quiet place where you can be alone.
2. Either sit or lie down in a position that is comfortable for you.
3. Close your eyes.
4. Take in three slow deep breaths. Focus on nothing but your breathing.
5. Bring your awareness to the top of your head. How does it feel? Are you feeling any pain or pressure?
6. Pull your awareness down over your face. Is there any pain in your sinuses? Is there any tension in your jaw?
7. Continue to bring your awareness lower. To the muscles in your neck and shoulders. Can you feel any tension? Stop for a moment when you get to your heart, and tune into the rhythm of your heartbeat. Keep going until you reach the bottoms of your feet.
8. Make a mental note as you scan down through your muscles, joints, and organs, if you think anything needs attention. Are you sitting too much at work? If so, maybe you could go for a walk at lunch or find a place to take a 10-minute stretch break in the morning and afternoon.

Take a 360 Body Check

Ask yourself how the other areas of the wheel are affecting your physical wellness. Here are some questions to help you get started, but you are not limited to just these questions. As you write and reflect, you may come up with more that are more personal for you.

360 Body Check Questions

(This will help you understand what could be causing the element of body to be out of balance.)

1. Are you eating foods that will help your body achieve optimal wellness? If not, what are you missing? If you are having a hard time answering that question, do you need an assessment and advice from a professional?
2. Are you getting enough sunlight?
3. How is the air quality in your home and workspace?
4. Do you take the time to breathe deeply at least once a day?
5. Are you allowing yourself enough time to rest? What does rest mean to you?
6. Are you drinking enough water? If not, how can you help yourself remember to do so?
7. Is your career taking a physical toll on your body? If so, how? How can you change or manage this?
8. Are your finances causing you stress, which in turn can be held physically in your muscles or cause you to breath more shallowly? This worry can also cause you to make poor decisions with your food. Take some time to really reflect on the physical implications your financial stress may be causing.
9. Are there any relationships in your life that might be compromising your physical health?

Your Mental State

There have been times when all areas of my life feel that they are in balance for me mentally. I wake up feeling focused. My thoughts are sharp. I can reason with more accuracy. And I can navigate my emotional state with more clarity.

Then there are times when my brain feels foggy. I'm unable to focus on the simplest of tasks. It feels like tasks that require even the most minimal amount of focus take so much time and effort.

I'm sure you've felt both of these times in your life as well. Of course, a lack of focus can sometimes be short-lived and based on a very surface level desire to not have to complete a task you don't want to. I'm not talking about that. I am talking about the longer periods when you get stuck in useless thought loops of worry, or your mindset is challenged.

Your Emotional State

Our thoughts drive our emotional state. Some of these thoughts we are conscious of, but some are embedded deeply in our subconscious and unconscious. How often do we have a knee jerk reaction to something but don't understand why?

Emotions! They drive us, but they can also be driven by us. Our mental state can affect our emotions and so can our physical state. Sometimes, though, our emotions can be the hardest layer of ourselves to maintain balance. We don't always understand where our emotions are coming from. There is so much to unpack and look through. From our spirituality to our connections with others, to the food we eat, it is all connected to how we feel and how we manage our emotions.

Our subconscious is a very powerful thing; so powerful, you may not even know when it is the underlying decision maker. Have you ever been so angry at a partner in your life for a seemingly small slight? When you look back on that anger in a moment of calm, you really aren't sure why you got so mad. In those moments, are you able to reflect? Are you able to be honest with yourself?

For your work in this section, you will begin by reflecting on this one very important question:

DO YOU LOVE YOURSELF, RESPECT YOURSELF, AND PRACTICE NO SELF-HARM?

Do you love yourself enough to make your wellness a priority over all else? Do you love yourself enough to get to know yourself on a deep level? Do you love yourself enough to figure out what your true purpose in life is? Do you love yourself enough to fight for that purpose?

When you love yourself, you work on yourself because your love calls for it. Love asks you to know yourself, to embrace yourself, and to surround yourself with everything that makes you feel good. Love asks you to achieve total health and wellness for yourself. You are the solution.

Moving Forward from Here

Stepping into the role of active self-manager is key to your wellness journey. It gives you the knowledge and strength to not only deal with but heal your chronic pain. Self-management is a decision you make for yourself to no longer suffer in silence. This book will guide you when it comes to some of the decisions you need to make. It will inspire you to get to know what your challenges are.

Wellness 360 Quiz

Go back to your Wellness Score. Which three areas scored the lowest for you? You can also pull from the reflections you've been doing throughout the chapter. Pick one to begin with.

As you know by now, this element has three components to it: a physical external layer, an emotional internal layer, and a mental symbolic deeper layer.

Ask yourself these questions related to the first element that is out of balance:

- The external layer of my _____element includes:
- One action step I can take to support my external layer of_____is:
- The internal layer of my _____ element includes:
- One action step I can take to support my internal layer includes:
- The symbolic layer of my _____ element includes:
- One action step I can take to support my symbolic layer is:
- What other elements of the W360 wheel might be affecting this element that is out of balance?
- What action step will I try in order to support this element, and when will I take this step?

Reframing Challenges

Now that you have a clearer idea of the challenges you are facing, you need to reframe them! Generally, when most people encounter obstacles, they tend to feel fearful and anxious. It's good to try to understand where that fear and anxiety is coming from.

One of my clients, Tim, was experiencing chronic knee and low back pain. He had his own business as a contractor and was finding it increasingly difficult to get into kneeling and crouching positions, due to his pain and limited movement. He was a year away from a potential knee replacement, but he was stressed and anxious about maintaining his function and work demands.

When we looked more deeply at the challenges he was facing, we explored alternate postures he could use at work. For some tasks, he began sitting on a low stool. He started wearing a knee brace. He also started to become more aware of reducing the amount of time he spent standing and maintaining prolonged positions. He learned about self-pacing techniques and was able to get through his days with more ease.

On closer examination, Tim also realized that he was slightly unsteady on his feet and needed to work on his balance through strengthening exercises. He began swimming and saw a physiotherapist who recommended the use of a cane. Although he didn't like using a cane, Tim knew it gave him the extra security he needed to do more.

Tim engaged in an active self-management program and sought out the help he needed. He recognized his challenges, he found solutions, and he sought help. This helped him to achieve his goals for his business, with less pain, and alleviate his anxiety about his knee surgery.

This is the type of active problem solving you need in order to achieve the goals you set out for yourself. With this in mind, add a few more questions to the list from above.

Let's look at some of the specifics of problem solving:

1. Decide on the top three elements that you feel are out of balance in your life.
2. Determine three problems in each area and how these problems impact your day.
3. Now determine what you would rather see happen with these specific problem areas.
4. What are the obstacles that are preventing you to reach these goals?
5. How are these obstacles impacting your life?
6. What would you rather see happen?
7. Make a list of some options that would solve the problem.
8. What are potential challenges that you could encounter with these options?
9. What are potential solutions to this?
10. Throughout this whole process, seek support and help.

In every aspect of your life, you should always devote more time to work on yourself than anything else. At the end of the day, it's all about you. Cultivate the energy you need every day to live in optimal health, and you will see growth in all elements of your life.

Chapter 3

Empower Yourself to Take Back Your Life

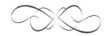

"Every human has four endowments—self-awareness, conscience, independent will, and creative imagination. These give us the ultimate human freedom... The power to choose, to respond, to change."
– Stephen Covey

The most important lesson you will learn in this book is: YOU ARE THE MANAGER OF YOUR LIFE. Yes, you are in control. You have the power to manage your pain. You have the power to heal. You have the power to take your life back! The time to do it is now, and I would argue that some of the most important work you will do on your journey to taking your life back will happen in this chapter.

No doubt if you are experiencing chronic pain, you may be feeling disempowered. You may be feeling removed from your own life. You may be feeling disconnected from yourself and others.

I found that some of my patients withdraw from life completely when they are feeling controlled by their chronic pain. They stop doing the things they once loved to do. In many ways, they stop living. On the flip side, I have had some clients who continue to live their lives in fulfilling and meaningful ways by finding different ways to do things. They find solutions.

The key is realizing what the problems are and finding ways to address them and set achievable goals. The difference with these two groups—the ones who stop living and the ones who embrace life—is not the pain itself but rather how they choose to manage their symptoms. Your self-management is always a choice, and if you choose to do nothing at all, this is still a choice.

The most important relationship you will have in this life is the one you are in with yourself. You need to be your own advocate. You need to be your own nurturer. Currently, there are aspects of your relationship with yourself that work, and aspects that don't. There are parts you are comfortable with and parts you are not proud of.

The best choice you can make for yourself is the one where you acknowledge and resolve the parts of you that are blocking you from growth, and nurture the parts of you that you are proud of.

Start Your Daily Success Journal

Daily Success Journal

I'm working on
this goal today

Purpose & Motivation

What is going to be
better when I have
reached my goal?

Power

What will I do today
in order to get
closer to my goal?

Focus

What is important
today?

Which of my core
values do I want to
focus on today?

Before we move forward into the work of this chapter, I want to share with you an invaluable tool that I use with all of my clients. It is a Daily Success Journal. It is so important for many reasons:

1. It allows you to see how far you've come. Sometimes, when you set goals and are slowly progressing with each day, it's difficult to remember where you started. It's easy to feel discouraged and give up when you can't see how much you've progressed. This daily success journal serves as a reminder of what you've accomplished on your healing journey.
2. Writing about your success is empowering. Each day when you sit down to think about how you've stepped up to take control of your life, you take pride in your work. The feeling of accomplishment pushes you to keep going, even when new challenges arise.
3. It provides insight into what works best for you and how to better advocate for yourself.

I can guarantee that this one tool will change your life for the better if you commit to doing it every day. If you miss a day, don't beat yourself up; just pick it up again the next day. Positive reinforcement and recognizing how much work you've done for yourself will be the fuel to keep motivating you on the days when you can't see the improvement.

I have created a printable PDF for you. It is right there for you to download and print at www.healyourchronicpain.com. I suggest getting yourself a binder and printing enough for at least 6 months. In a way, you are writing the journey of your success from this day forward!

Focus on the Solutions

As we talked a lot about in the last chapter, identifying the challenges you are facing is the first and most important step to finding effective solutions.

Sometimes we are not directly aware of how we are contributing to a challenge. It is in understanding this that you begin to figure out what you need to overcome it.

Generally feeling a sense of uneasiness in the body is a good sign. It warns you that you might be putting yourself in harm's way. When this becomes a problem is when you use this feeling to get in the way of doing the things you love in life, or even pushing harder to take control of your life. Sometimes it's easier to give into the feeling and not try, than it is to find a solution, but often this can be more detrimental to your healing journey.

Here is an example of what I mean:

Melissa is a patient of mine with multiple sclerosis. She is usually quite upbeat and was very disciplined in maintaining the goals she set out for herself. One day, she showed up for a session looking unhappy and defeated. When I asked her why, she responded by telling me she wasn't quite sure why she felt this way. On deeper probing, she realized that it was because she had been asked by some friends to join them on a trip to Portugal. Normally, an opportunity like this would've excited her. But with her MS, she was worried that she would hold her friends back. The thought of being a burden really bothered her, even though her friends had promised that they didn't mind pacing things for her. They really wanted her to come.

Melissa knew that no matter what, there would inevitably be a lot of walking on the trip, and this was her main challenge. What if she couldn't keep up with their slower pace? What if her friends got frustrated with her? What if they regretted asking her on this trip and never asked her again?

Even though Melissa had made great progress and was consistently succeeding at achieving her goals, the thought of not being able to go travelling because she didn't have the physical endurance was a big blow. It made her feel powerless. Subconsciously, it made her wonder why she was working so hard.

As she shared, I asked her to remember back to her success journals. She took it out of the bag she always carried with her, and she read about some of the moments that had made her most proud. The most impactful memory was the day she decided to take control of her MS and live a full life that she loved. With this in mind, and some renewed determination, we began to brainstorm some solutions to Melissa's challenge, which was the issue of endurance.

Here are a few of the solutions she came up with in our discussion:

1. *Get a really good pair of comfortable walking shoes.*
2. *Use walking poles.*
3. *Rent a Segway or an e-bike.*

With each new idea, Melissa felt a renewed excitement about the trip. She decided that she would rent both an e-bike and a Segway prior to the trip to test them out and see if they were viable options. This is important. It's great to have a solution in mind, but you always have to make sure they work first. if you miss this step, you'll be setting yourself up for failure. If none of your options work, then it's time for you to seek more resources.

The great news for Melissa is that she was able to combine the use of good shoes, walking poles, and an e-bike in Portugal. Her friends were so glad she came and were happy to take time to rest when she needed it. She never once felt like a burden, and she was so glad she identified the challenge she was facing and found solutions rather than letting it stop her from living life.

Commit to Yourself & Have Faith

"Until one is committed, there is hesitancy, the chance to draw back.
The moment one definitely commits oneself, then Providence moves too.
All sorts of things occur to help one that would have otherwise
never have occurred. Whatever you can do, or dream you can,
begin it. Boldness has genius, power, and magic in it."
– Johann Wolfgang Von Goethe

Being diagnosed with a chronic condition that results in pain can be frightening. It has the ability to take away your sense of security, safety, and control. You could also experience shock and trauma when receiving a potentially life-altering diagnosis. You could feel some uncertainty about the future and your ability to continue to do the things you want and like to do.

Many find it difficult to make decisions when faced with uncertainty and doubt. One of the hardest tasks that effective self-management will ask you to do is to not let your doubt get the better of you.

The flip side of doubt is faith. Doubt scatters and disseminates your energy, whereas faith solidifies it. When I mention faith, I don't necessarily mean a faith in God, but rather faith in yourself or something bigger than yourself. Faith is not a belief; it is the willingness to accept reality as it is and also to accept the unknown. Faith creates a willingness that is needed when your willpower is struggling in the face of things that are difficult, demanding, or boring.

Faith is a recipe made up by three parts: trust in yourself; an understanding that although you don't know the outcome, life will work out; and an intuitive connection with your higher self.

So, commit to yourself and have faith that you too can succeed. Once you've done this, you can begin to take action. Faith is a quiet cousin to courage. Your faith will give your courage what it needs to follow through with the decisions you need, to achieve your goals based on your values.

We have discussed how to identify your challenges, and the importance of identifying exactly what your obstacles are, so that you can find effective solutions. This is great but it's not complete. This has to be followed through by action. When this action is empowered with faith and your "why," you can achieve anything you set your mind to.

Make a Decision Already!

First of all, make a decision to commit to yourself! Make a decision right now to explore your values, understand your why, and create smart goals based on what you know you want your life to be.

Making decisions and seeing them through is also a very important tool in your self-management. Life is full of decisions, with some of them being much easier to make than others. When you are feeling indecisive about something, it can get you down. When you feel like you don't know what to do, it can have a negative impact on how you are feeling.

Having good decision-making skills is something your life can only benefit from. Here are some tips to help you decide what to do when you feel like you can't figure out a plan:

Don't let stress get the better of you!

Avoid making a decision at all when you are stressed. Make sure you are feeling calm and open minded. Stress can put you off your game and may increase your stress response. What is a stress response? I'm sure you know what it is, because I'm sure you've had more than one in your life. It's that moment where you make a flash decision based on the negative emotions you are feeling due to a stressful situation.

If you're feeling anxious about a decision, try to manage your stress so that it doesn't cloud your thinking. It's your willingness to want change here that is more important than your willpower. If you think that you don't have the capacity and energy for the change, becoming aware of the change you need and why is a tool to fuel your willingness. When you decide there is something you need to do, it's important to know *why* you are doing it. Your *why* is connected to your set of core values and beliefs. Knowing why we do something is an important tool. The why is the reason behind an action; if the reason we do something is not connected to what we deeply value, then we wouldn't be successful in that action. The "why"—the reason we do something—is a catalyst like a fire stick to our transformation.

Often, I ask clients what their *why* is, and most often they cannot answer. When you don't know why you are doing something, it generally is because you are making a choice based on someone else's value system. Knowing YOUR core values empowers every decision you make. It aligns you with how you feel and think. When you follow through on these decisions with action, then you are on the path to living each day in alignment. Aligning with your value system is such a powerful tool in intention setting, because it connects you to what you deeply believe. When you choose your actions based on your core being, you are living in a natural state of l**oving** what you are doing. This is key, **loving what you are doing**, because when things get tough and your willpower is waning, then a willingness over willpower wins this battle every single time. ***Knowing your "why" comes from your core values, and this is key to goal setting and making decisions.***

Here are a few easy ways to manage your stress, especially if you need to make a decision that will impact your life:

1. Sit and focus on your breathing. Breathe deeply. Allow yourself to become aware of your breath and nothing else.
2. Go for a walk. Turn your thoughts to the beauty of the world around you.
3. Find support. Talk to a family member, friend, therapist, coach, or healthcare provider.

It's so important to manage your stress, especially when you are making a decision about a stressful situation.

Give yourself time to think and space to breathe.

Give yourself the chance to sit with a problem for a while so that you can process your options and feel comfortable about the course of action you choose.

Identify what you want based on your goals and values.

Be true to yourself. Be true to what you value in life!

Identifying your values helps you to make a decision that feels right, and to stick to it. When you factor into a decision the things that are important to you, the best option will, more often than not, become obvious. At any rate, you're more likely to end up with an outcome you're happy with. The change you seek might be small or big; but whatever it is, the transformation you need is deep, and it's easier to choose when you understand yourself. With the knowledge of what is driving you, you can make more informed decisions that will ultimately make your life better.

Your Values Will Help You Decide

> *"There is only one corner of the universe you can*
> *be certain of improving, and that is yourself."*
> **– Aldous Huxley**

The only way to improve your life is to understand your values. When you make decisions based on what you value most in life, rather than depending on external sources to tell you what you value, then you will make decisions based on those values. These decisions will help you improve yourself, your outlook on life, and how you feel about each day.

Values are essentially what all people seek to one degree or another. Values have been categorized to help you understand what your values are:

- **Physical values include** food, survival, safety, shelter, heat, and protection from the elements.
- **Mental values include** security, freedom, independence, and health.
- **Emotional values include** peace, happiness, harmony, balance, and satisfaction.
- **Higher level values include** self-expression, contribution, purpose, creativity, and spiritual connection.

These only include some of the possible values that could be most important to you. There are more than a hundred of them, and they continue to grow as humanity does. Your values will also grow with you. If you're having a hard time defining yours and need a list of values to help you get started, go to www.healyourchronicpain.com to check out the downloadable version I share.

Be Like Melissa

Let's take a moment to think back on Melissa's story. She recognized that there was something bothering her, but she didn't know what. She then identified a challenge. She came up with some possible solutions. She made a decision, she sought resources, she assessed her options, and she then successfully achieved her goal.

On the following page are a few more tips to help you with your decision-making skills so that you too can achieve the success Melissa did.

Identify your options.

Making a decision can result in several different outcomes, and not all of them may be obvious. When considering each option, don't just list the positives and negatives; write down any likely consequences.

Weigh your pros and cons.

When faced with a big decision, sometimes we lose sight of the big picture. Write a list of pros and cons for each course of action and then compare them. Sometimes the cons aren't nearly as bad as we imagine them to be, or the pros might make your options more obvious.

Talk it out.

It can be helpful to get another person's perspective on your issue, particularly if they've faced a similar decision in their own life. Sometimes, as we saw in Melissa's case, talking it out can help you get to the root cause of the issue and help you come up with options.

Plan how you will tell others.

If you think someone may have a bad response to your decision, think through what their reaction is likely to be. Put yourself in their shoes to help you think of a good way to manage the situation.

Setting Your Goals

Before you take meaningful action, you must determine what you want to achieve and why. Have you heard of SMART goals? Have you ever created a goal and couldn't figure out why it was so hard to achieve? Sometimes goals are set and they are simply unachievable because they aren't clearly measurable; for example, "My goal is to feel better." How can you achieve this goal without really defining what it means? How do you measure it? Goals can also feel unattainable if they have no deadlines attached to them; for example, "I aim to be a writer one day." If there's no urgency, this goal will never make it to the top of your priority list.

When you set your goals, make sure they are SMART:

SPECIFIC AND MEASURABLE: If your goals aren't specific and measurable, you have no way to track them and, therefore, no easy way to measure your progress. This means you often forget about your goals or lose motivation. Bottom line: Your goals never actualize.

ATTAINABLE: Attainable goals are ones that challenge you but aren't unreasonable. For instance, if you haven't exercised in a while, make your goal something like walking or biking for 20 minutes a day. Don't make your goal to be to "run on the treadmill for 45 minutes." The first is a challenge; the second is unrealistic. The first gives you a chance for success; the second sets you up for failure.

RELEVANT: Making goals that are relevant simply means making goals that are meaningful to you. Don't create the goals you think you should have, or go online and list goals that other people have (unless they truly inspire you). Instead, create goals that are right for you, ones that align with your values and priorities.

TIME-BOUND: This step simply means putting a time frame on your goals. For example, don't just write, "I want to exercise more." Write, "I want to exercise three times a week." A time frame creates motivation and makes your goals trackable.

Take a moment now to write out a list of your goals.

Evaluate Your Goals

I know this process can seem overwhelming if you've never done this before, but I promise it's not. Investing the extra time to make good goals can be the difference between you achieving them or not.

Have a look at each one and assess whether or not it is a SMART goal. Ask yourself:

1. Is it specific?
2. Is it measurable?
3. Is it attainable? (Keep it challenging yet reasonable.)
4. Is it relevant? (Is it important to you in your life now?)
5. Is it time-bound?

Put a star beside the goals you want to start with.

Let's look at another example for more clarity:
Let's say one of your goals for the year is "to take better care of yourself." This doesn't give any specifics on what taking better care of yourself actually means to you. Does "taking care of yourself" mean eating better? Does it mean taking more time for relaxation? Does it mean getting active? Define what self-care means to you and create SMART goals that will help you take better care of yourself.

For example:
1. *My goal is to be active every day. I will go for a 20-minute walk every day and take a yoga class at least twice a week.*
2. *My goal is to learn to meditate. I will begin by reading one new book on meditation a month. I will find a guided meditation to help me get started, and for the next month, I will meditate for 5 minutes every morning.*

It's tough enough to simultaneously work toward your many goals while also keeping up with everyday life. If your goals are not crafted to set you up for success, you're likely to lose track of them before too long. And you'll probably rewrite that same goal next year. You can prevent this by making it SMART to begin with. Once you do that, you have helped yourself to become organized and accountable.

Mind-Mapping

When brainstorming my goals, I like to use another tool called mind-mapping. When creating yours, use any method that works best for you. Here I start with my original goal.

For an example:

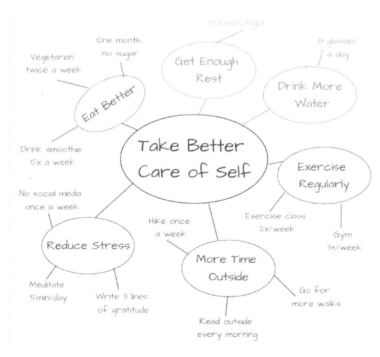

There are many ways to reach any specific goal. As you can see in the above diagram, your job is to list the options and then choose one or two to try out. If this is hard to do on your own, seek help from friends, family, a coach, or healthcare professionals. It is important to have a list of options, but eventually you will have to prioritize and try the ones that you feel are most promising.

Take Action

Once you have identified a goal and created a list of ways you might achieve this goal, you now have a plan!

The thing with goals is that they often feel like dreams: You think about them, you envision them, but sometimes they still feel unattainable.

The secret is to not try to do everything all at once. Do one thing every day that will move you forward. I don't mean that you don't do anything else, but choose one thing that gets your energy and attention for that day. Look at how much you can realistically achieve in a week, and create an action plan that is doable. An action plan is for the short term and will evolve as you evolve. This is you designing your road map toward achieving your goal.

Action plans are a great self-management tool. They allow you to plan and implement the things you know you require to do in order to attain your ultimate goals. Your plan needs to be action specific; and again, it has to be measurable. Remember the examples from above.

It's not enough to say you want to exercise more. Get specific about your plan by asking the following questions:

* What are you going to do?
* How much will you do?
* When will you do it?
* How often will you do it?

Rules for creating a successful action plan:

- It is something you want to do.
- It is achievable (able to accomplish in that week).
- It is action specific.
- It answers the questions of what, how much, when, and how often.
- On a scale from 0 (not at all sure) to 10 (absolutely sure), you are confident you will complete your plan at a level of 7 or higher.

Implementing Your Action Plan

Successful action plans are about writing a plan, tracking how you are doing, and checking off what you were able to do. If you are not able to tick things off your list, then maybe your plan was not realistic. Only by tracking this are you then able to problem solve the roadblocks you encounter.

And remember those Daily Success Journals? Now is the time to start using them. Even if your goal was to simply finish this chapter and develop your goals, start writing about your achievements. Pat yourself on the back. You've started!

Check In

At the end of each week, check in to see if you are closer to accomplishing your goal. Taking stock is a very valuable step. You may not always notice daily progress, but you should see a little progress each week. If you notice that you are not reaching your goal, then it is time to revisit the goal with problem solving skills or with the help of a coach.

Expect Midcourse Corrections

To end this chapter, I want to share with you one last concept that is so important to achieving success: mid-course corrections. Expect them and embrace them!

When you are trying to overcome obstacles, your first plan may not turn out to be the most effective one. Expect that you will need mid-course corrections. Don't give up when things aren't working; keep an open mind and try something else. You can also give yourself more time to accomplish difficult tasks, or modify the steps in your short-term action plan.

- You are here.
- You know your values.
- Your goals are set.
- You have a plan.
- Take action!

Chapter 4
Navigate Your Nutrition Now

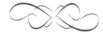

"Healthy eating isn't about counting fat grams, dieting, cleanses,
and antioxidants; it's about food untouched from the way
we find it in nature in a balanced way."
– Pooja Mottl

You are what you eat! I'm sure you've heard that saying more than once in your lifetime, but it always bears repeating. The food you consume is an essential player in your health journey. Eating healthy simply means that **most of the time** you make good and healthy food choices. It does **not mean** being **rigid or perfect**. No matter what the media or your friends say, there's no one best way of eating that fits everyone; there is no perfect food.

When it comes to your health and eating, it's easy to forget that you are a unique being. In your quest to eliminate chronic pain, you assume the latest fad diet advertised must be the answer. You might think to yourself, "If it worked for my friend Mary, then it will work for me. And if my co-worker can lose 10 to 20 pounds by eating nothing but cottage cheese, so can I."

When the peanut butter and celery diet fails, you are left wondering what went wrong. But the next day, there is a new diet to try, and so you jump back on the roller coaster. When I learned to stop blaming myself, I figured out the truth: There is no diet that will work for everyone. Always remember that the best tool you have is your body's own wisdom. Yes, the answer to why and how to eat lies within you, not on the cover of your favourite magazine.

The human body is a complex and marvelous machine, much like a car. A car needs the proper mix of fuel to run right. Without it, your car may run poorly and could even stop working. The human body is similar; it needs the proper mix of good food, which is its fuel.

Can a car run on empty? NO! Neither can your body; and just like a car, it will also begin to run poorly if given the wrong fuel. Healthy eating cuts across every part of your life. It is linked to not only your body's health but also your mind's well-being.

When you give your body the right fuel and nourishment, here's what happens:

- You have more energy.
- You don't feel tired in the afternoon.
- You increase your chances of preventing or lessening health conditions such as heart disease, diabetes, cancer, and some chronic pain conditions.
- You feed your central nervous system and brain, which can help you handle life's challenges as well as its emotional ups and downs.

The work you are about to do in this chapter will help you understand how your current eating habits may be a detriment to your health, and how to shift into a healthier way of looking at food.

Diets Don't Work

I know from years of working with my clients on their eating habits, and from my own personal experience, that DIETS DON'T WORK. Yes, you might see some people achieve success through dieting, but more often than not, people fail. Why? There are three main reasons why diets don't work:

- They don't address the fact that your body is unique and therefore has it's own unique set of needs.
- They are extreme.
- They are often too restrictive for the average person. Diets set people up to feel like failures because, inevitably, people will break and have some of the food they've been depriving themselves of, which makes them feel like they can't do it.

I used to be a yo-yo dieter until I discovered that there is a much better way. There was a period in my life where I thought I was healthy. I was running marathons and still couldn't take the pounds off. The way I thought about food and how it was being used to fuel my body was all wrong.

The way you fuel your body is unique to you and dictated by your nature. Of course, we all know that if you want to lose weight, you need to be cognizant of the amount of sugar and calories you eat each day, but this isn't what it's all about. You should never approach an adjustment to your diet from a place of deprivation. You are never going to maintain a perfect diet. Let yourself have some of those things you enjoy, like chocolate, but do it in more of a mindful way.

Generally, when you eat the good stuff, your body feels better, and you feel better. Let's go back to the idea of what this means for you specifically. When it comes to food and my health, I follow an ancient Indian science called Ayurveda. According to this science, there are three different body types, or doshas. Your dosha is based on your constitution. The three doshas are Vata, Kapha, and Pitta. To learn more about these and take the quiz to find out if you are one of these or a combination of them, visit my webpage (www.healyourchronicpain.com).

The more knowledge you have, the better prepared you will be to fuel your body in the most effective way for you. You are unique. Your body is unique. Your life is unique. No healthy eating plan should follow a cookie-cutter formula. The one thing to remember as you read through this chapter and begin to come up with a plan that works best for you, is that your body holds all of the answers you need. Listen to your body. Be open to understanding what it is telling you.

Have you ever eaten a big lunch that was delicious, but you felt tired and needed a nap almost instantly? What was your body telling you here? A lot of people joke about having a "food coma" after a filling meal, but it's not a joke. It's your body's way of telling you that the fuel you just gave it made it feel lethargic, and therefore didn't provide the energy you need to have a productive day.

65

Listen. Listen. Listen. Your body is constantly communicating with you! One of my wellness coaching principles I learned is that your body is a laboratory. There are three main ways it gives you messages about the fuel it needs. We talked about the first one in the last paragraph. Your energy levels are a great indicator. Sometimes, other than feeling tired, you have a burst of energy that doesn't last long. This is again another indicator that you haven't given it the right fuel.

The second way it communicates is through the symptoms you might feel, like a gassy stomach or the burn of acid. The third way is through cravings. You might suddenly crave some red meat, which isn't normal for you. Or you'll just know that a piece of fruit is what you need to lift your energy and help you focus. All of these signals are your body's way of helping you come up with a healthy eating plan.

Begin to see your body as your friend, and think of this project as a collaboration. The Wellness 360 way of achieving holistic health will help you look at food and your body differently.

Journal Your Food Truth

> *"When diet is wrong, medicine is of no use.*
> *When diet is correct, medicine is of no need."*
> **– Ayurvedic Proverb**

Before we continue on in our learning, I want to inspire you to get started with your food journal. I know. This is not always easy, and many of my clients have found it to be a very annoying task, but I promise you it is absolutely necessary. You may think you know what you are eating daily, but it's not as accurate as you might think. When you write it down and can look back on an entire week of what you've eaten, it is eye-opening.

One of the biggest benefits of journaling, especially for anyone with chronic pain, is that it helps you understand what foods are working against you. Yes, your food sensitivities can be making your pain worse! When you are writing in your journal, note if your pain, symptoms, emotions, or mood got worse after a meal. *NOTE: If you suspect some foods are a problem, eliminate them one at a time to test your idea. Again, it is important not to eliminate entire food groups. Always eat a balanced diet of fruits, vegetables, grains, proteins, and healthy dairy choices. And don't forget to hydrate.*

Make a commitment to yourself in this very moment, to complete a food journal for as long as it takes you to understand the kind of fuel your body needs in order to operate at optimal health. Remember that the connection between food and energy and overall well-being is incredibly powerful—just by changing the way you eat, you can radically change the way you look and feel and think.

A few easy steps to get you started with your food journal:

- Buy a journal that you like and will inspire you to write, or open a new document on your computer.
- Make time each day, just a few moments, to sit and record the food you've eaten.
- Find a quite space where you won't be interrupted.
- Don't judge yourself or edit. Be truthful.

There is a downloadable link for you on my website, www.healyourchronic pain.com.

What Is Healthy Eating?

At the heart of healthy eating are the choices we make in the long run. Healthy eating is being flexible and allowing yourself to occasionally enjoy small amounts of food that may not be so healthy. There is no such thing as a perfect eating style. Being too strict or rigid and not allowing yourself to ever have treats will likely cause your best efforts to fail.

If you have chronic pain or other conditions, healthy eating means having to be somewhat choosey about the foods you eat. For example, some people with migraines need to avoid certain foods that might trigger a headache. People with diabetes need to watch their carbohydrate intake to manage their blood sugar levels. They do best by deciding which carbohydrate rich foods (fruits, bread, cereals, rice, etc.) they will eat each day. People who are at risk for heart disease can control their blood cholesterol levels by controlling the amount and kinds of fat they eat. Consuming the right amounts and types of fat can also reduce inflammation for some kinds of chronic pain conditions.

Those with high blood pressure can help lower it by eating lots of fruits, vegetables, and low-fat dairy foods. For some, cutting back on salt lowers high blood pressure. And to maintain, lose, or gain weight, everyone needs to pay attention to how many calories they eat.

The real issue for most of us is not the healthy foods we consume but the less healthy ones. One-third of most North American diets are made up of foods that are high in added sugars, solid fats (butter, beef fat, pork fat, chicken fat, stick margarine shortening), and salt. The North American diet also tends to contain a lot of food that is made from white flour and other refined grains. These added sugars, fats, and salt contribute to high blood pressure, diabetes, and obesity. There's evidence that an unhealthy diet may be associated with chronic pain as well.

Trade-offs are a big part of healthy eating. This means learning how food affects you and then deciding when you can treat yourself and when you should pass. For instance, it may be important to you to have a special meal on your birthday. If so, then you can make healthy food choices when you're out for casual lunches, on days that are not special occasions. Trading off like this can help you stay on the path of healthy eating. It gets easier with practice, and it even becomes part of your everyday life.

A good starting place is to move toward eating more plant foods: fruits, vegetables, whole grains, legumes, nuts, and seeds. This does not mean giving up meats and foods that may be high in sugar, fat, or salt, but rather eating them in smaller amounts or less often.

The goal is to maintain a healthy balance in the kinds of foods you eat and how much you eat. That all sounds simple, but every day, we are faced with hundreds of food choices. It is often easier and quicker to grab something less healthy than to give more time and thought to what we will eat. So how do we put together meals that are tasty and enjoyable and yet healthy?

The 5 Key Principles of Healthy Eating

1. **Choose foods as nature originally made them.** This means the less processed, the better. By processed, I mean foods that have been changed from their original state by having ingredients added (often sugar, salt, of fat) or removed (often fiber or nutrients) to make them taste better.

2. **Get your nutrients from food, not supplements.** For most people, vitamins, minerals, and other dietary supplements cannot completely take the place of food. Unprocessed foods contain nutrients and other healthy compounds such as fiber, in the right combinations and amounts.

3. **Eat a wide variety of colourful, minimally processed foods**. Your goal is to get more variety, more colours, and fewer processed foods on you plate. These three simple rules will give your body all the good things it needs. Think blue and purple for grapes and blueberries; yellow and orange for pineapple, oranges, and carrots; red for tomatoes, strawberries, and watermelon; green for spinach, kale, and green beans. Don't forget the white and warm brown tones from mushrooms, onions, cauliflower, and whole grains such as brown rice.

4. **Foods high in phytochemicals**. Phytochemicals are compounds that are found only in plant foods—fruits, vegetables, whole grains, nuts, and seeds. There are hundreds of health-promoting and disease-fighting phytochemicals in the unprocessed foods we eat.

5. **Eat regularly.** A gas-fuelled vehicle will not run without the gas, and a fire eventually burns out without more wood. Your body is much the same. It needs refueling regularly to work at its best. Eating something, even a little bit at regular intervals, helps keep your "fire" burning. Eat at regular times during the day, preferably at evenly spaced intervals. This helps maintain and balance your blood sugar level. Blood sugar is a key player in supplying the body, especially the brain, with energy. If you do not eat regularly, your blood sugar drops. If it becomes too low, it can cause weakness, sweating, shaking, mood changes (irritability, anxiety, or anger), nausea, headaches, or poor coordination, which can be dangerous for many people.

Learn How the Food You Eat Can Help Ease Your Chronic Pain

"The doctor of the future will no longer treat the human frame
with drugs, but rather will cure and prevent disease with nutrition."
– Thomas Edison

If food can give us energy or take it away, and if food can make us feel sick or make us feel better, then why can't it help alleviate chronic pain? The short answer is that it can. When you eat for your body's needs, you help give it the fuel it needs. For the remainder of this chapter, you are going to read about some of the tips and tricks that will help you eat your way to better health, even with chronic pain:

• Know the must-have brain boosting super foods the body needs to promote self- healing.

- Learn about the connection between food and your mood. Help yourself choose foods for renewed energy, vitality, and self-nourishment.
- Overcome stress eating, eating out of boredom, and eating unconsciously.
- Identify your food sensitivities. These trigger your specific symptoms.
- Learn easy tips to overcome a sugar addiction. Eating less sugar will eliminate the extreme highs and lows in your energy levels.
- Understand common challenges you might face when making healthier food choices. This will help you identify your pitfalls and learn strategies to overcome them.

Eat Yourself to Energy

There is a very simple, easy trick to help you feel less tired and increase your energy throughout the day: Eat good food! There are certain foods that work to keep your blood sugar levels steady. The best part is that they can be tasty and easy to integrate into your everyday diet! These superfoods help to recharge your internal batteries and give you more long-term energy. I am going to share a couple of them with you in this chapter, but if you want to access the full guide I've created with all 25 super foods, there is a downloadable PDF on my website (www.healyourchronicpain.com).

#1 Cocoa
Qualities:
- Boosts energy
- Enhances concentration
- Lifts mood
- Balances blood sugar levels
- Helps kick addictions
- Increases supply of oxygenated blood
- Promotes liver health

Cocoa is one of the richest sources of antioxidants. It contains chemicals that can help to ease depression and the symptoms of stress. Buy a brand that is unsweetened, 100% pure cocoa powder.

It's rich in:

- **Magnesium** – Encourages energy, reduces sluggishness, and addresses mood swings.
- **Iron** – Necessary for the production of oxygen-carrying red blood cells.
- **Anandamide** – Raises levels of serotonin, endorphins, and dopamine, all of which help you to relax and lift your mood.
- **Flavonoids** – Help to reduce insulin resistance and stabilize blood sugar levels.

#2 Kale

Qualities:
- Balances blood sugar
- Boosts production of red blood cells
- Raises energy levels
- Supports liver function
- Promotes health of the adrenal glands
- Regulates hormones
- Helps overcome addictions
- Boosts immunity

One study found that eating a diet rich in vitamin E, of which kale is a great source, reduces the risk of developing diabetes by about 30%. Avoid eating in large quantities if you have an under-active thyroid gland.

It's rich in:
- **Calcium** – Encourages restful sleep and aids in nerve function.

- **The B vitamins** – Eases fatigue, anxiety, and depression, and boosts concentration and energy levels.
- **Iron** – Encourages the production of oxygen-carrying red blood cells.
- **Vitamin C** – Boosts immunity, helps to prevent damage to cells as a result of stress, and encourages a healthy metabolism.

Eating for Your Mood

"Your diet is a bank account. Good food choices are good investments."
– Bethenny Frankel

Do you eat when you are bored, sad, or feeling lonely? Many people can find comfort in food. They eat when they need to take their minds off something or have something else to do. Some people eat when they're feeling very anxious, angry, or depressed. At these times, it is easy to lose track of how much you eat. It is also easy to make unhealthy choices when you're feeling this way. Here are some awesome ways to help control these urges:

When you feel the urge to eat, ask yourself if you are really hungry. If the answer is *no,* make yourself do something else for 2 to 3 minutes. Go for a short walk in the house or around the block, work on a jigsaw puzzle, brush your teeth, or play a computer game.

Keep your mind and hands busy in your downtime. Getting your hands dirty is always helpful! Try gardening for some fun.

If you can't stop yourself from reaching for a snack because you are bored or procrastinating or feeling anxious, reach for celery sticks or an apple. If you are reaching for a fun snack to treat yourself, why not try popcorn instead of chips and fatty dip.

As we talked about earlier, keep a food journal every day. List what, how much, and when you eat. Note how you are feeling when you have the urge to eat. Try to spot patterns so that you can anticipate when you want to eat without really being hungry.

Write down action plans for adjusting your eating habits, like the ones we talked about in Chapter 3. Reading these will help you handle it better when you feel like eating based on your emotions. Your daily success journal (which is different from your food journal) is very important here to keep you on track, and I can't emphasize that enough!

Here are some tips to help you overcome emotional eating and reconnect with food that will help you stay happy and energetic:

- **Slow down when you eat.**
  If your excuse is that you were too busy to slow down for eating, consider the adage, "You can't pour from an empty pitcher." How often do you find yourself saying that you are too busy? Is it so often that your life's manta is, "I'm too busy?" First, you need to change that mantra. Consider that the world is not as fast paced as you think it is. By changing your belief about the world, your view of your own life will change. Begin to imagine that your world is slower, and take time for stillness. When you begin to experience stillness throughout your day, your body will thank you. Most people avoid stopping to reflect because they are fearful of what they may discover within themselves. When you step out of your daily routine and take even just a moment for peace, you allow your body's wisdom to speak up.

- **Pay attention to what you are eating.**

- **Get your senses into some mindful eating.**

- **Chew your food.**
  If this sounds insignificant to you, think again! If you come to the table in a rush, your body will remain in the stressful state of the fight or flight response. Imagine your body as it tries to digest food, thinking that it is

going to fight a war. Your body will choose to store the food for later, and that's how all of those extra pounds are packed on! Chewing your food allows your digestive juices to do their job by helping you properly assimilate food and absorb nutrients. Also, chewing your food and experiencing the taste, texture, and smell of each bite will lead you to a more enjoyable experience. When you relate with your food in this way, you will be less likely to go looking for something else in the pantry an hour later. Saliva releases enzymes that help break down food. You should chew each bite 50 times. Take a bite and mindfully chew. You'll be amazed to discover that the more you chew, the more flavor your food releases!. For your information, 70% of the human immune system is located in the gastrointestinal tract! That's why proper digestion is the number one key to vibrant health.

- **Eat and listen.**
  This is not your everyday food journal. Keep a log of what you eat every day and how you feel two hours after eating it. Are you still hungry? Are you too full? Are you satisfied? Is your stomach settled? What are you craving? By listing not only what you were eating but also how it made you feel, you will begin to make a connection between what you eat and how it affects your digestion and your energy levels. Do you want to learn how to turn on your inner radar so that you can listen to what your body is telling you? Most importantly, you will create the mind-body connection that is often missing in today's dining experience.

- **Honour your body.**
  Start by making your health and your body a priority. Try a new exercise routine, go for a brisk walk, or participate in a yoga class. When you take time for your health and well-being, you send positive messages to your body. Begin to talk to your body, and eliminate the negative messages that you subconsciously send to it.

Try this exercise. Begin by standing in front of the mirror naked—yes, that's right. Stand there for five minutes and notice what you love about your body. Then state it out loud. Repeat this several times a week until you feel connected to both your physical and emotional self. When you concentrate on the beauty that you have, you will, by law, attract more beauty. When you slow down, chew your food, eat and listen and honour your body, you will reconnect with that inner voice that tells you each day all you need to know about what to eat, when to eat, and how much to eat. There is no one single miracle diet that will tell you what your body needs in order to be happy, fulfilled, and healthy. You are your own guide to healthy eating and living.

- **Feed your spirit.**
  If you're lonely, bored, hate your job, are nervous or grieving, haven't healed your emotional wounds, have a spiritual void, or feel uninspired by your exercise routine, you may eat simply as a psychological attempt to fill the void in your life. No amount of ice cream will ever soothe the sting of your parents' harsh words. However, journaling or counselling will. If this is why you experience cravings, take a good, long look at your life and make the appropriate changes to fulfil your soul. Happiness does not come from food; it comes from within.

Sometimes we sabotage our happiness from a super subconscious and erroneous belief that we don't deserve the very, very best in life, and we compensate by eating downright poisonous foods such as fast-food French fries or an entire bag of potato chips. We may likewise indulge in junk foods when we are feeling particularly healthy and fit. Then our body responds with low energy levels, mood swings, or getting sick, so we repent for our guilt of being happy.

- **Conscious eating.**

  Do you find that you are often doing other things while you eat? Are you watching TV or standing over the sink talking on the phone? It can be strange; you may not even be hungry, but every time you do a certain activity, you are looking for something to munch on. This happens because the mind begins to associate the two activities. For example, whenever you watch TV, you may feel like you want to eat something. The TV also helps to disconnect your mind and your hunger from one another, and suddenly, before you know it, you've eaten the whole bag of cookies even though you weren't even hungry.

  Your body wants to be present with food and really experience it. You actually digest the food more efficiently when you are focused on eating. How can you be more present when eating?

Steps to intuitive eating:

- Make a conscious choice to eat.
- Ask your body what it wants to eat. Your logical mind might jump in at first, telling you what you should or shouldn't have. It will take a little practice to understand what your body is telling you. But you'll see how your intuition will talk to you with food.
- Eat with awareness. Be present when you eat. Notice the texture and the taste of the food. Chew it, and sit down while eating.
- Eat the entire experience, not just the food. Food is more than just about putting it in your mouth. It's also about the preparation—the thought you put in, the smells as it's cooking, and the time it takes. Everything is a part of your eating experience. That's why, when you eat fast and all of a sudden, it's gone, you find yourself wondering where it went, because you haven't allowed yourself to truly experience the food you've made. Soon

you find yourself hungry again, but what you are hungry for is the experience of nourishing yourself, rather than the food itself.

- Listen for feedback. After you eat, take a few minutes to relax, and reflect upon what you've eaten and how you ate it. How do you feel? Are you finished? What would you do differently next time? Then, let it go. After you finish, forget about food. Humans are notorious for thinking about what they ate for hours, feeling guilty for bad choices, and thinking about what they will eat next. Do something you enjoy instead that has nothing to do with food.

You Will Face Challenges

"If you keep good food in your fridge, you will eat good food."
– Errick McAdams

As you know, food has the ability to make you feel better, but if you are eating the wrong foods for all of the wrong reasons, it will only make you feel worse—physically, mentally, and emotionally.

Improper eating habits according to Ayurveda:

- Overeating
- Eating soon after a full meal
- Too much water or no water during a meal
- Drinking very chilled water during a meal or, indeed, any time
- Eating when constipated
- Eating at the wrong time of day, either too early or too late
- Eating too much heavy food or too little light food
- Drinking fruit juice or eating fruit with a meal
- Eating without real hunger

- Emotional eating
- Eating incompatible food combinations
- Snacking in between meals

When you attempt to change these habits, you will face challenges. These things are ingrained in your daily life, and some of them are attached to strong emotions. Go easy on yourself. Remember, your journal is your friend in this. Write about what you're eating; how you're feeling, both emotionally and physically as you shift your patterns; and of course, write down your successes.

One of the big challenges you might face is an addiction to sugar. This is very common! Here are some tips to help you quit your sugar addiction:

- fruit and sweet veggies. Not only will this help you get your five to eight servings of fresh fruits and vegetables daily, but it will curb your sweet tooth!
- Drink plenty of water. Sometimes having a sweet tooth is a sign of dehydration. When the sugar bug bites you, drink an extra glass of water.
- Use natural sweetness. Maple syrup, honey, and brown rice syrup are downright miraculous.
- Incorporate spices. Sweeten your foods naturally with wonderful spices such as cinnamon, vanilla, nutmeg, cloves, coriander, or cardamom.
- Reduce or eliminate caffeine intake.
- Get plenty of sleep and rest.
- Reduce the amount of animal foods in your diet.
- Eliminate low-fat or prepackaged foods.
- Indulge in the SWEET MOMENTS rather than sugar! Get plenty of hugs from family and friends, read a good book, go on an adventure, or watch the sunset. When you regularly enjoy life's sweet moments, you naturally reduce your need to medicate with refined sugar.

Another common complaint I hear from my clients when they are attempting to eat healthier, is that the food just doesn't taste good anymore. Here are a few pointers to help your food always taste delicious:

- In cooking, use herbs like basil, oregano, and mint, and spices like cinnamon, cumin, curry, ginger, nutmeg, and turmeric, or sprinkle them on top of food when you're ready to serve.
- Squeeze fresh lemon or lime juice on foods.
- Use a small amount of vinegar on top of hot or cold foods. There are dozens of choices, from balsamic to berry and fruit-flavored varieties. Experiment with new flavors.
- Add healthy ingredients to the foods you usually eat (carrots or barley to soup, for example, or dried fruits and nuts to salads), to give them more texture and make them tastier.
- Chew your food slowly and well. This will allow the food to remain in your mouth longer and will release more flavor.
- If the lack of taste is keeping you from eating enough, you may need to add more calories to your meals or snacks.

For many of my clients, they feel that by the time they've finished making a meal, they are too tired to eat. Here are some hints to help:

- If you do have energy, cook enough for 2 to 3 or even more servings of meals, especially if it's something you really like. Freeze the leftovers in single serving sizes.
- Do a meal exchange with friends or family; freeze what you receive, in single serving sizes. When you are tired, choose one of these precooked meals to reheat and enjoy.
- Break your food preparation into steps, resting in between.
- Ask for help, especially for big holiday meals and family gatherings.

- Do a relaxation exercise about half an hour before mealtime, or take time out for a few deep breaths during a meal.
- Prepare food that is easy to eat, such as yoghurt pudding, or a drink, such as a protein shake or a fruit smoothie.

Arm Yourself with as Much Information as You Can!

The more you know, the better off you will be, especially when faced with challenges. I know how hard it can be to change your eating habits. The last section of information I want to share with you is a list of useful Ayurvedic tips to aid with digestion. These are incredible, and I use them every single day!

- Eat half a teaspoon of fresh grated ginger with a pinch of rock salt before each meal to stimulate digestion.
- Salt also aids digestion and helps to retain water.
- Alkalization helps digestion and regulates gastric digestion
- This stimulates digestion and improves digestion.
- Small sips of warm water during a meal will aid digestion and absorption of food. Do not drink ice water as it slows down the digestive fire. Indeed, ice water should not be taken under most circumstances, as it is too shocking to the system.
- Proper chewing is essential to good digestion, ensuring food gets thoroughly mixed with saliva. SLOW DOWN WITH EATING.
- A cup of lassi/kefir at the end of a meal also aids the digestive process. Make by blending a quarter cup of yoghurt with two pinches of ginger and cumin powder in 1 cup water.

Ideally, you should fill the stomach with 1/3 food and 1/3 liquid—1/3 should remain empty.

Eating for Your Health Is a Choice

Healthy eating is about the food choices you make most of the time. It is never about being able to eat certain foods. There's no such thing as a perfect diet. Healthy eating means enjoying a moderate amount of a wide variety of minimally processed foods, while allowing for occasional treats.

Eating this way will help you maintain your health, prevent future health problems, and manage your pain condition symptoms as best as possible. Think of changing your relationship with food as doing something positive and wonderful for yourself, not as a punishment. It is the ultimate in self-care! As your own self-manager, it's up to you to find the changes that are best for you. If you experience setbacks, identify the problems and work at resolving them. You can do it! I am here to help.

Here is a full list of the tools I provide on my website (www.healyour chronicpain.com), which will help you establish a better relationship with food:

- List of brain boosting foods, with easy recipes to make your meal planning easy.
- List of foods that create inflammation, which you can use to identify your food triggers.
- List of foods to substitute for sugar, so that you never have to take the sweetness out of life, and you can continue to find enjoyment in your food.
- Quiz to get to know your specific constitution so that you can make choices to increase your capacity to heal.
- Information on emotional hunger, along with a "Feelings Worksheet" from the IAWP.

Chapter 5

Move Mindfully
Toward Better Health

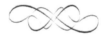

"Nothing happens until something moves."
– Albert Einstein

W hen there are restrictions in how you move, I think you can agree that you don't feel great. The simple fact is that when you change how you move, you will change how you feel.

Active people are healthier and happier than people who are not active. This is true for people of all ages and conditions, including chronic pain. Not moving enough can cause or worsen pain, disability, and other illness. In order to better manage your chronic pain, you need to learn how to balance activity and rest. Equally important is planning for regular activity and exercise.

Physical activity keeps you fit so that you have the strength, stamina, and energy to do the things you want to do in life. Being more active can improve your chronic pain over the long run. Scientific research conducted over the past 30 years has consistently shown that increasing physical activity helps ease chronic pain, improve function, and boost overall health and well-being. In fact, exercise is most often the largest part of rehabilitation programs for people with chronic pain. The bottom line: ***Keep moving!!***

You probably know that regular physical activity is important, but when you have chronic pain, it can be difficult to know what you can do and how to do it in a way that won't hurt you more. The good news is that there is plenty of information available to help you get started and be successful.

In this chapter and the one that follows, you will learn about these guidelines and how to make wise exercise choices. Of course, learning what to do is not enough—you have to do it! Your life is your responsibility. It is up to you to make your days more enjoyable, more comfortable, and healthier through physical activity.

As is the case in every chapter, the information about exercise in this book is not intended to take the place of medical or other health professional advice. If you already have a prescribed exercise plan that differs from the suggestions here, be sure to share this book with your healthcare provider and therapist before beginning this program.

Be Open

"Healing is more about accepting the pain and finding a way to peacefully coexist within it. In the sea of life, pain is a tide that will ebb and weave, continually. We need to learn how to let it wash over us, without drowning in it. Our life doesn't have to end where the pain begins, but rather, it is where we start to mend."
– Jaeda Dewalt

Don't be afraid to open yourself up and try something new. Fear is there to protect us, but it can also keep us stuck. Take time to look at your fears and ask yourself what may be keeping you stuck.

Consider things such as:

"I'm afraid I can't keep up."
Or
"I'm afraid I'll make a fool of myself."
Or
"I don't know how to use the machines. I hate asking for help."

Keep in mind that fitness is a journey, not a destination. If you're afraid you can't keep up, start slowly until you get stronger. Safety comes first in every situation.

Many people hold a preconceived notion that the gym is filled with people with perfect bodies. This simply isn't true. People visiting the gym, and even those holding gym memberships, are just like everyone else whose goal is to live a healthy and balanced lifestyle. Even if you're really out of shape, don't worry about it and don't obsess over your appearance. You'll find many supportive people every place you go.

The bottom line is, don't be afraid to put yourself out there and be the real you. Never forget that you're not alone. Most importantly, go at your own pace and be safe! Asking for help and assistance is a sign of strength, not a sign of weakness. Don't hesitate to ask a gym employee or trainer for help. That's what these people are there for and they are happy to assist you. Most likely, they're cheering you on each step of the way!

Open yourself up to living a more healthy, mobile lifestyle by recognizing your fears and then letting them go. It's okay to be afraid, but it's not okay to let it hold you back from living a happy life.

Write a Letter to Your Fear

Sometimes it can be hard to vocalize your fears. You might not be able to put it into words, or you might feel silly, or you may worry that others just won't understand why you feel so afraid and will not take you seriously. A great exercise that I have found to be so helpful, not only for myself but also for my clients, is to write yourself a letter about your fear. This allows you to feel more in control of your fear, rather than letting it control you.

Here are a few tips to help you get started:

1. Grab your journal or your computer, whichever you feel most comfortable with. Find a quiet place in your home where you won't be disturbed.

2. Don't edit! Just let the words flow. Leave your judgements out and be kind to yourself.
3. Write about what your fears are and where they are coming from.
4. End your letter with a promise to yourself to not let these fears hold you back.

What Do You Already Know?

You know more than you think you do. Take a look at your past experiences. What do you already know about your relationship to exercise? In other words, what worked for you in the past, or what didn't work for you? Then ask yourself, "Why was I so successful at this?" Or, "Why didn't this work for me?"

Knowing the answers to these questions is a first step in determining where you want to go from here. Remember, if you keep looking, you will eventually find exactly what you're looking for and precisely what you love. Sometimes, the answer has been there all along.

What's Your Excuse?

This question can be an even harder one to address than what your fears are. This requires you to be accountable! When you allow your excuses to get in the way, this is honestly on you. Sometimes your excuse is fear, and if that is the case, then you need to recognize those fears and work through them. Go back to the letter exercise. Sometimes it is you finding reasons to not do something you don't want to do.

If you find yourself making excuses not to move your body, you may not have found your exercise "joy." Take notice of when you find yourself making excuses about your exercise routine.

Some of your excuses may include:

- I'm too tired to exercise.
- I have too many things to do; I don't have time.
- I'm too old to start exercising.
- I'm not athletic and I'm overweight.
- I don't have the right outfits or clothes to start exercising.
- Exercise is boring.
- The kids have homework and I need to make sure they get it done.

If you find yourself making excuses, look for ways to turn these excuses around. For example, if one of your excuses is that exercise is boring, find activities you love to do. If the gym makes you feel confined to small spaces, try taking a walk in nature. If there isn't a trail available to you, look for a track at your local high school. There are often many walkers on the track after school has let out for the day, doing exactly what you're looking to do.

If you find yourself saying that you're too tired to move, go for shorter, lower impact intervals of exercise you really enjoy. This is a great way to motivate yourself and fit some exercise into your daily routine.

It's true that our children oftentimes have a bountiful amount of homework in hand when they come in the door after a long day at school. Children, however, need a break too. Taking a fifteen-minute family break and playing tag or walking the family dog is a great way to spend time together as a family and get in some much-needed movement. Enjoy your time together and find creative ways to get your body moving.

My main message here is to stop letting your fear and excuses get in the way of moving. There is always a solution. Make incorporating exercise into your daily schedule and you will find the excuses falling away.

Why Exercise?

Exercise is the key to a healthy life. With movement, you can help in the management of heart disease and diabetes. It improves blood pressure, blood sugar, and blood fat levels.

Here are a few more benefits to regular exercise:

- It helps you maintain a good weight, which takes stress off your weight-bearing joints.
- It is also part of keeping bones strong and treating osteoporosis.
- There is evidence that regular exercise can help prevent blood clots, which is one of the reasons it can be a particular benefit to people with heart and vascular diseases.
- Regular exercise improves levels of strength, energy, and self-confidence.
- Regular exercise also lessens feelings of stress, anxiety, and depression.
- It can help you sleep better, which allows you to feel more relaxed and happier.
- Regular exercise has consistently been shown to be the single most important thing you can do to manage chronic pain.
- It improves the ability to do normal activities by reducing pain, tenderness, and fatigue, while increasing muscle strength in people with various types of widespread pain, including fibromyalgia.
- It lessens pain and improves function in people with chronic back pain.
- Strengthening and stretching exercises improve chronic neck pain and some types of headaches.
- Strong muscles help people with arthritis to protect their joints by improving stability and absorbing shock.
- Regular exercise also helps nourish joints and keeps cartilage and bones healthy. Many people with pain from poor circulation or other causes can walk farther and more comfortably with a regular exercise program.

This is all good news! But the best news is that it doesn't take hours of painful, sweaty exercise to achieve health benefits. Studies have shown that even short periods of moderate physical activity can improve health and fitness, lessen pain, improve everyday functioning, reduce disease risks, and boost mood. Being active also helps you feel more in control of your life and less at the mercy of your chronic pain! This last benefit is a big one:

•   **REGULAR EXERCISE ALLOWS YOU TO TAKE CONTROL OF YOUR LIFE!**

The Ayurvedic Approach

Now that you know what's been holding you back, why exercise is so important, and that you have some life experience that will give you a starting place in your fitness journey, let's look at another tool you can use to understand the type of movement that works best for your body.

Body Typing

Knowing how our own body works can help you feed it, like we talked about in the last chapter, and take care of it through exercise, in ways that it will respond best. Many cultures have found ways to categorize the body in different ways to help humans understand how to help themselves feel good and live longer.

We can distinguish how our bodies differ by blood type, metabolism type, personality traits, and by many other methods. While there are a variety of body type theories, one of the oldest and most predominant comes from Ayurveda. The science of Ayurveda is over 5,000 years old and originated in India. Ayurveda means the "science of life" ("ayur" meaning life and "veda" meaning science). Traditional Chinese medicine, Tibetan medicine, and early Greek medicine all have links to Ayurvedic concepts. While many see it only as a system of healing, it is truly a way of living that provides daily guidelines on diet, exercise, behaviour, and overall health.

Each person has a unique combination of the three body types, called doshas, defined in Ayurveda: Vata (wind), Pitta (fire), and kapha (Earth). This unique combination shapes our physical body and mental and emotional characteristics. Identifying a person's dosha provides clues to how he or she can balance themselves, both physically and psychologically. If you haven't already, please refer to the dosha quiz on my website: (www.healyourchronic pain.com).

It may seem strange to you to look to a system of defining body types to figure out the best exercise for you, so I wanted to share some of the examples listed by the IAWP, based on the Ayurvedic body typing:

Large-framed, endomorphic, Kapha

Aerobic: starting slow, moving up progressively to vigorous exercises – walking, jogging, dancing, sports, and anything promoting perspiration

Thin, undernourished, ectomorphic, Vatta

Aerobic: easier, gentler, low-endurance exercises like yoga, walking, hiking, biking, and some jogging; avoid a routine that tires or stresses them out

Muscular, mesomorphic, Pitta

Aerobic: encourage those of Kapha, but with moderation and for purpose of stress relief; enjoy cycling, mountain climbing, hiking, swimming, and more extreme sports; avoid excessive competition

They provide more options for stretching and strengthening your body, as well as how to take of your body post-exercise. Download the full list from my website.

Yoga for Better Health & Awareness

"From Asana arises steadiness of body and mind,
freedom from disease and lightness of the limbs."
– Hatha Yoga Pradipika 1.17

Throughout my life, I have tried many different forms of exercise. I love moving! But it wasn't until I found yoga that I began to truly listen to my body with an authentic awareness. For me, it is so important to continuously explore the connection between the body, mind, and soul; and yoga has provided the perfect way for me to do that. Yoga had been a part of my life for a long time, but after deciding to become a yoga teacher, it has grown to have a very large place in my daily living. I do feel that it has everything, and that is why I am going to focus a large portion of this chapter on why yoga is the complete package.

Although understanding body mechanics and physical alignment through posture is so important, there is something to be said for emotional alignment as well. When I work with my clients, I always highlight just how important it is to pay attention to the spiritual. You are a full package and every part of you is connected. The one thing I know yoga does is that it inspires an exploration of that connection, and rather than compartmentalizing the body for physical fitness, it brings in the whole person.

I will begin by sharing some information on yoga postures or Asanas. They are one of the most important systems of physical culture ever invented; but that said, I want you to keep in mind that yoga is about so much more. Most people in the West perform Asanas as exercise. This has become the meaning of yoga for them, which they associate with yoga postures. While Asanas can be a discipline in their own right, also known as exercise or therapy, it should not be confused with the role of Asana in classical yoga, which goes beyond this.

Asanas reflect an amazing understanding of how the body works and, in particular, how to release tension at a deep level from the tissues, organs, and joints. Asanas keep the body in the best possible health. They provide specific positions and movements designed to strengthen and stretch the musculature, which can effectively move the body away from pain and illness, toward more balance in the body. They keep the spinal column subtle in order to create the optimal flow of energy through the nerves that innervate the organs and glandular systems. And, perhaps most importantly, they begin a systematic cleansing of the tissues, preparing the body for deeper yoga practices.

Asanas are a part of a sacred science that comprehends all aspects of consciousness. They make up one step in the eight-fold path of yoga and prepare us for pranayama, breathing, and meditation. They reflect not only a profound knowledge of the body but also of prana (life force energy), mind, and spirit, of which the body is only an external image or manifestation.

Here are the eight steps of yoga as outlined by Patanjali:

1. Guidelines for interacting with others
2. Niyamas – Guidelines for interacting with yourself
3. Asanas – Physical postures and techniques
4. Pranayama – Breathing exercises and techniques
5. Ptrayahara – Giving your five senses a rest
6. Dharana – Focus and concentration on a single point
7. Dhyana – Experience of meditation
8. Samadhi – Experience of your true nature

How to prepare yourself for a yoga class:

*   Yoga is ideally performed on an empty stomach with the bladder and bowels evacuated. Try to wait at least three hours after eating before performing yoga, and empty your bladder before the practice. The Asanas

involve deep organ level stretching that promotes intense circulation; we must empty the bowels to avoid circulating those toxins.

- It is also best to bathe before yoga to remove dirt, sweat, and other toxin buildup from the skin. The original practice of yoga is gentle and does not create much sweat, so after practice, you can continue on with your day.
- The best time I find to practice is in the morning after I wake up and before breakfast, but if this doesn't suit your schedule, you could practice at any time during the day.
- If you're menstruating, you may want to encourage downward flow, rest, and reflection, and avoid inversion poses and intense stretches. This might also be a time when you increase the meditation component of the related relaxation part of your practice.
- When you begin your practice, set a positive intention that will help carry you through your practice and help set a tone for your day.

Examples:

- I can heal myself.
- I am supported.
- Life force energy is abundant and all around me for me to receive.
- I am fully present.

The premise of yoga is that it should be comfortable, not painful; pleasurable, not competitive; and focused on inner joy rather than comparison to others. At different times of the day, on different days, and at different times in life, our bodies will have different capabilities, so we must be compassionate with ourselves while practicing yoga. It is not a practice of pushing past physical limits and pain, but rather working within a physically comfortable practice that helps us indirectly push through mental limits and strengthen our spirits. So only do what is comfortable for your body, even if it is just a slight movement toward the full pose; you should only feel a healthy strain in your body. "No pain, no gain" does not apply in yoga!

As you schedule your practice, you should plan enough time to end with a calm relaxation pose, a period of meditation. Whether or not you choose to perform meditation, conclude your practice with a deep chant. After you complete your practice, you want to avoid eating heavily, drinking anything stimulating, or engaging in any vigorous activity. Allow yourself to stay in a calm state. Try to leave a gap of about 10 to 15 minutes in this state to enjoy the results of your practice.

Benefits of Yoga

Once you get going with a regular yoga practice, you'll start to see all kinds of benefits showing up in your life. Lots of research studies have been undertaken to show how yoga can truly benefit different aspects of health and wellness.

Here are a few benefits of yoga you can look forward to in your regular practice:

- **Greater flexibility.** This is the most obvious benefit that most people are aware of. Flexibility is good for preventing injury and giving you better control over your body. You'll feel great!
- **Less anxiety and depression**. The mindfulness aspect of yoga can help calm an anxious mind. It can also bring a feeling of greater peace, which can decrease depression. This benefit will carry you through your day, bringing a great sense of wellness into your everyday life.
- **Increases body awareness.** When you move unconsciously, you are more likely to get injured. Yoga teaches us proper posture and conscious movement.

- **Releases tension.** Yoga teaches you to calmly lean into specific poses and to breathe while holding the pose. This encourages your muscles to relax and release, which can seriously reduce tension.
- **Helps with sleep**. The calming aspect of yoga, physical nature of the poses, and mindfulness practice can help you when it comes time to go to bed.
- **Improves balance.** Many yoga poses depend on you maintaining your balance while holding the pose. This is a great way to strengthen your body and gain greater control of your muscles and coordination.
- **Increases blood and lymph flow.** The various poses in yoga have you twisting, turning, and even going against gravity. This is great for massaging the circular and lymph systems, pushing blood and lymph fluid around. From Downward Dog to headstands, you'll find a pose that can help create better circulation in your body and warm up those hands and feet.
- **Improves posture**. Each pose that you do in yoga requires proper posture for it to work. That means that you have to consciously think about the way you're holding your body, for almost an hour or more. Over time, you'll find your posture-related muscles have strengthened and you're holding your body in better form.
- **Improves focus and connection.** Do you ever feel like your body is in Canada and your mind is in England? Yoga can help you connect your body and your mind while helping you focus on the moment.

Focus on What You Love

I know I've spent a lot of this chapter focusing on yoga, and I am willing to admit that yoga is my choice because I have felt the benefits in my own life and witnessed it in countless clients. That said, you ultimately have to choose what you love.

If you hate going to the gym, you most likely won't be able to maintain a gym membership and get the most value for your money, no matter how good it may be for you. On the other hand, if you love nature and being outdoors, hiking and playing tennis may be the exact exercise program you're looking for. Design your life and build your exercise routine around the activities and places you love and enjoy.

Wellness 360 Body – The Symbolic Layer

Our body on a symbolic layer represents alignment. Some questions to consider as you explore this layer are:

- What does alignment mean to you?
- How does your internal world match your physical world?
- How aligned are you internally with what you desire externally?
- Does your external reality match up with your internal intentions?
- Are there any unexplained physical manifestations that may be related to being out of alignment?

Our bodies often show symptoms related to being out of alignment in some way. For example, a person might have lower back pain if they are experiencing stress about their finances, relationships, or career.

Whenever you examine this third layer, because it's more of an invisible layer, you want to ask yourself if any part of you is resisting this element. If your body is out of balance, alignment is affected. What part of you is resisting this element? It's a simple question, but it can trigger you to look deeper at why you might be out of alignment in the element of body.

Remember that a Wellness 360 approach to your body means that you don't just take a pill to fix your pain. Instead, you look at each of the element's layers to really understand from a holistic perspective what is happening both inside and out and how you can support your body.

Why does body alignment matter to your health?

It's definitely important to focus on eating well and exercising, but that's not all there is to wellness. To be truly healthy and experience well-being, you must address all areas of your life. You want to understand the areas of your life that are causing you stress, and work to decrease that stress to find balance. Only then can you thoroughly create alignment in your body.

You can feel the effects of the things you are struggling with by how much your chronic pain is bothering you, or by the well-being (or lack of) expressed on your face. You might also feel how well your life matches up with your desired life by how aligned you feel in your body.

Create Body Alignment in Your Life

The body holds the keys to uncovering the things in our lives that need attention the most. By tuning in, we can better understand what is going on in our minds at a subconscious level. You might struggle to really understand why you feel the way you do. But by spending time deeply embodied, you might discover insight that you won't find from the external world. Your body is wise and willing to help you toward even better levels of wellness.

Here are a few ways to begin to create more bodily alignment so that you can deepen your well-being:

Create an embodiment practice.

Our culture spends way too much time in our heads. We value logic, reason, and thinking over almost all other qualities. Our jobs are very brain-centric, and our social system is set up to prefer using our minds almost exclusively. So, we get out of touch with our bodies and don't understand how to interpret what our bodies are trying to communicate. We develop pain and even more disconnection.

99

An embodiment practice is one path that can help you get back to being in touch with your body. It can be any type of movement that works best for you. Yoga, tai chi, or any slow, gentle movements are all great options for practicing embodiment. The key is to do something that engages your body, pulls you out of your mind, and pushes you into just feeling your body.

Start a regular mindfulness practice.

To go with embodiment is deepening your experience of being out of your mind and into your body through mindfulness. While yoga and tai chi can help create space for mindfulness, you don't need to be moving to get deep into these healthy spaces.

Mindfulness is a perfect place to meditate on your body and re-learn how to listen to it again. You can start with short sessions of quiet or try out a guided visualization specifically about drawing your consciousness into your body. You might even be able to find a local meditation class that is focused on this specifically.

Be patient and stick with the process. After your practice is well established, you'll see all kinds of wonderful health benefits. Plus, you'll start to have moments of wisdom that help you know how to direct your life toward more well-being.

Journal about alignment in your life.

Writing down your thoughts in a mindfulness practice sort of way can be really helpful for uncovering how you truly feel. Ask yourself some hard questions about your life:

- Do you say what you mean?
- Do you do what you say you are going to do?
- Are your relationships in alignment with who you are inside?
- Do issues in your life (such as your finances or career) align with who you want to be?

- Are you engaging in behaviours that are red flags that something's off (binge eating or drinking, insomnia, avoidance when things matter, etc.)?

This doesn't need to be done all in one journaling session. It's a good idea to let yourself gently explore your mind, heart, and body through these questions, picking up sensations, intuitions, and nagging feelings. Trust yourself to know how to help yourself heal. Be brave enough to face the things you're avoiding. Heal the things that you know you're ready to heal. Your journal is a great place to start uncovering these healing journeys.

Commit to self-care.

People have a tendency to get really busy and then avoid taking care of themselves. Does this sound familiar. You run yourself ragged, racing here and there, never really slowing down to find out what you need. When you do this, you tune out physical pain and symptoms, you ignore relationship issues, and you keep your mind busy so that you don't have to face the struggles.

When you commit to caring for yourself, however, you commit to slowing down enough to check in often. Show up for yourself. Take the time to eat well, engage in daily movement, get enough sleep, attend healthcare appointments, and share quality time with the people you love. Life is never perfect, which means you don't have to wait until it is, to start doing wonderful things for yourself.

Align yourself to care for your body.

Creating alignment in your life means creating alignment in your body. The reverse is also true. When you focus on more alignment and well-being, you'll create a happier life and a healthier body. You'll feel more joy, peace, and calmness. Life will feel easier, and you'll feel more confident in it. You're worth this kind of care, and it's never too late to get started. Tune into your body, find out what it's telling you, and then do the work needed to heal.

The Bottom Line

Physical activity is a great path to feeling better and finding balance, both in your health and in your life. As a general goal, aim for at least 30 minutes of physical activity each day and commit to doing it every day.

If you want to lose weight or meet specific fitness goals, you may need to exercise more. Remember to check with your doctor before starting any new exercise program, especially if you haven't exercised for quite some time, have chronic health problems such as heart disease, diabetes, or arthritis, or you have any other health concerns.

Chapter 6

The Art of Breathing for Chronic Pain

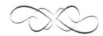

"Why do you stay in prison when the door is so wide open?"
– Rumi

You probably don't think much about breathing, mostly because you don't have to. This autonomic reflex occurs in healthy adults whether or not we consider what's going on when we inhale or exhale. The breath is a remarkable tool we can use to heal a variety of conditions. Breathwork for chronic pain is just one way you can use your own body to heal itself. In this chapter, I am going to help you get started with your own breathwork practice.

My journey into exploring pranayama and breathwork techniques, as shared by the ancient Rishis, has been a deeply profound journey. This quote by Rumi captures exactly the essence of what I am attempting to share with you.

Breath is the essence of life! Your breath supports every experience you have, from the time of your first inhalation to that of your last exhalation. In yoga, the breath is intimately associated with prana, your life force energy. Learning to regulate your prana to calm, balance, cleanse, and invigorate your body/mind is a powerful technique in yoga.

The study of the benefits of breathwork is a relatively new field. Laypeople are not the only ones to take breath for granted; researchers have also not paid much attention to the value of deep, even breathing when it comes to our overall health and well-being. However, the field of research is catching up. Major studies are beginning to illuminate the benefits of breathwork and have found these key insights:

- Deep yogic breathing alleviated major depression in patients who were previously unresponsive to treatment.

- Breathing therapy works better than cognitive behavioural therapy to reduce panic and anxiety.
- Rhythm of breathing affects memory and fear.
- People with severe PTSD, who are unable to regulate their breath, benefit from device-guided breathing (essentially, guided breathwork).
- Studies of veterans with PTSD have also shown that breathwork stimulates the vagus nerve, which helps to calm and quiet racing thoughts and anxiety.

Over the next chapter, I'm so excited to share my experience and teachings with you. Understanding how a breath practice can help you manage your chronic pain is a powerful tool that you can use every single day, not only in your physical healing journey but in your spiritual and emotional ones as well. My wish is that you will explore this deeper with me now, and then continue to explore this on your own.

Breathing & Chronic Pain

Physically, chronic pain is not simply a symptom. It is an illness. Emotionally, chronic pain decreases your ability to process clearly because it increases your anxiety and depression. Socially, it causes to you to retreat from the world, making you feel alone.

Breathwork is one of the greatest tools you can master, to help you not only physically manage your pain but cognitively manage your emotional and social responses. When you are living in a state of constant pain, it can affect your breathing, taking away the quality of the life force energy you are able to share with all of your cells. You can change this. You can take your breath back and give your body what it needs. Move through your pain to a healthier and happier version of yourself. Your breathing can affect your thoughts and emotions; therefore, when you take the time to breathe intentionally, you can affect how you live your life. You can help yourself to develop more positive thoughts surrounding yourself, your relationships, and your life.

What is breathwork?

The term "breathwork" or pranayama techniques simply means using conscious breathing techniques; and in the case of chronic pain, using it therapeutically. The practice goes back thousands of years to the ancient Rishis of India and is referred to more traditionally as pranayama. Pranayama is a Sanskrit word that combines "prana" (energy) with "yama" (control). The practice of pranayama is simply the control of our life force energy through breathing.

In yoga, pranayama is the practice of moving energy through the energetic channels of the body. This yogic practice of breathing is one of the eight limbs of yoga. In yoga's eight step path, pranayama is the fourth step. The ancient yogis have shared with us in great detail ways to improve and maintain our life force energy, the breath being only a part of pranayama techniques used. There's so much depth and wisdom in these teachings, and these pranayama techniques are the doorway between cleansing and energy work attained during the Asana (yoga postures), which then take us closer to deeper states of meditation.

The goal is to bring more energy to the body and to use the breath therapeutically (more below on the types of breathwork). Scientifically, when you inhale, your diaphragm moves downward to make space for breath to enter your body. This also opens the chest cavity to make room. As you exhale, the diaphragm moves up, pressing breath back out of the body.

When you focus on breathing slower, longer, and smoother, you activate the vagus nerve in the parasympathetic nervous system. The vagus nerve reaches from deep inside your belly, all the way up to the base of the brain. Our parasympathetic nervous system is a "rest and digest" system, only active when we are relaxed and at ease. Breathing lowers cortisol and adrenaline production to encourage the body to relax.

Whether you call it pranayama or science, the idea behind breathwork training is to use the breath to focus the mind, calm anxiety, and fully oxygenate the body.

Breathing Meditation:

Take a break from your reading here to begin your breath practice. I am purposely asking you to give this a try at the beginning of the chapter, so that you can take note of how much your breathing will change as you gain more knowledge and awareness. Try this:

- Sit quietly, uninterrupted.
- Close your eyes.
- Inhale deeply.
- When you reach the top of your inhale, begin to exhale slowly through your nose (like you are exhaling through a straw, connecting the inhale and exhale without a space.
- If your mind is racing or unfocused, picture a peaceful place or a time when you felt good/happy and serene.
- Continue connecting your inhale and exhale, going deeper each time, connecting without pause.

By practicing breathing meditation, it will become easy to apply during stressful events. If you have pain or an ache, send healing to that spot with each inhale and exhale. Ahhhhh.

How Could Breathwork Help with Your Chronic Pain?

Remember when you were little and scraped your knee so badly that the skin came away and pain started immediately? Chances are that fear of the

108

accident that caused the scrape, combined with pain, made your breath short and shallow. Maybe you cried so hard that you had trouble catching your breath, even forgetting about it until a caregiver reminded you to breathe.

Breathwork for pain is the grown-up version of comforting that small child in pain. And it works.

Research on pain perception and mood has found that deep and slow breathing reduces autonomic activity (the fear-based, fight-or-flight response) and pain scores. Another study found that pain scores in women with fibromyalgia decreased drastically in a cascading effect. The more pain decreased, and the more they kept breathing deeply, the more pain decreased.

Even when chronic pain alters a person's physiology, breathwork for pain relief is effective. One study of patients with chronic lower back pain and altered core muscle activation and breathing patterns, found that breathwork significantly decreased pain.

And when pain levels do not decrease as a direct result of breathwork, other research shows there is still an improved quality of life in chronic pain sufferers. Why? The deep breathing helps patients to better cope with the stress and anxiety that often surrounds dealing with a chronic condition.

The mechanism behind breathwork for chronic pain is not well-understood. Breathing does not remove pain, necessarily, but it does alter a person's perception of it. Practically speaking, better oxygenation of the blood improves healing, and lowers levels of cortisol and adrenaline, allowing your body to rest and relax instead of tensing with pain.

In essence, breathwork changes not only your perception of pain, but also your body's response to it.

Breathwork & Your Brain

The brain has many components, but in our present stage of evolution, we are only able to utilize some of these. This means that there are areas of the brain that we are attempting to awaken and integrate into our consciousness. In order to awaken dormant areas of the brain, we must spread the prana into these dormant areas, because the part that is illuminated or lightened is but a small fragment.

In your daily life, you mainly use the frontal lobe of your brain; however, underlying this is all the unconscious activity that you are unaware of. Pranayama is so powerful because it helps you develop the relationship between the unconscious and conscious brain. It brings the conscious part of the personality into contact with the unconscious part.

At the base of the brain is the structure called the reticular activating system. It is from the reticular activating system that energy arises upwards and awakens functions in other parts of the brain. Above this is the medulla oblongata, which contains the respiratory centres, and then there are the limbic systems and the hypothalamus gland, which controls fear, rage, blood pressure, hunger, satiety, weight control, pleasure, sexuality, and other functions. The structures that control respiration exist in the base of the brain, and it is this part of the brain that we are able to influence by using breathwork techniques. Of all the unconscious automatic and autonomic nervous system processes in the body, the only one that can be consciously controlled is breathing.

Your breath has control over all other internal processes of the body, such as the heart, digestion, blood pressure, excretion, and absorption. By developing a relationship with the conscious part of the breath, we are able to influence the deeper and more subconscious aspects of the consciousness. Your breath should be considered an instrument, to cultivate different states in the body. When learned to be used effectively, it can be the most fantastic and powerful instrument. Breathwork is called pranayama in vedic science, and the practice of yoga is aimed toward realizing this.

Breath Is the Essence of Life

You inhale for the first time; Prana is certainly superior to hope.
Everything rests on Prana.
Prana works through its own Power.
Prana gives Prana to Prana and Prana directs Prana to Prana.
Prana is the father, Prana is the mother,
Prana is the brother, Prana is the sister,
Prana is the teacher,
and Prana is the Brahmin.
– Chandogya Upanishad verse
Translation by Swami Lokeswarananda (obtained from Akhanda yoga)

You inhale for the first time when you enter this world. From that moment on, you take approximately 17,000 breaths each day, which over a lifetime total about 500 million breaths. In your final moments on this planet, you exhale for the last time; that breath defines the end of your life. Breath is your constant companion, silently and constantly taking in oxygen and expelling carbon dioxide, without a conscious thought needed. Your breath supports every experience you have, from the time of your first inhalation to that of your last exhalation. Breath is life.

In addition to keeping you alive, your breath also helps you move, think clearly, and control your emotions. For example, in intense moments, your breath automatically quickens. Calming your breath in these moments helps you calm your thoughts, which helps you respond to the situation more rationally. Yes! There is a direct connection between how you breathe and your emotions. Ask yourself these questions:

- How do you breathe when you are happy?
- How do you breathe when you are sad?
- How do you breathe when you are angry?

- How do you breathe when you are anxious?

It has been proven that by manipulating the breath, you can directly affect your emotions and feelings. This happens because you can hack your nervous system with the breath; thus, you can effectively use your breath to move from a sympathetic, flight or fight response, to a parasympathetic response, rest and digest state.

Your State of Mind Reflects the Quality of Your Life

Active breathing is said to have a very subtle influence on your level of consciousness. People who have a larger lung capacity can send oxygen around the body faster. You could increase your lung capacity with yoga and breathwork techniques that have been passed down to us from the ancient yoga tradition.

Your breath integrates many layers of your life: your environment, your respiratory tract, your nervous system, your mind, and every cell in your body. Regulating your breath enhances your physical, emotional, and spiritual well-being. It is the key to a healthy, vibrant life. For most people, breathing is the only autonomic nervous system function that they can influence.

Modern physiology divides the nervous system into two main components: the voluntary nervous system and the autonomic nervous system. The voluntary nervous system is active when you clap your hands, wave your arms, or use your legs to walk. It is responsible for activating the muscles that form the hundreds of facial expressions you make in a day, as well as those that control your speech. Although many of these functions occur with only minimal conscious intention, you have the ability to initiate and stop the use of these muscle groups as well.

The autonomic nervous system governs basic bodily functions, which you usually have no conscious ability to influence. These include physiological functions such as heart rate, blood pressure, regulation of your temperature and the levels of hormones in your body, perspiration, and the movement of food through your digestive tract. Your autonomic nervous system also plays an important role in the regulation of your immune system. Modern neurological signs suggests that most people are incapable of directly affecting their physiological processes. They function on their own whether or not you're paying attention to them or attempting to alter them.

Most people do not know how to influence their blood pressure, change the flow of the blood, reduce the sweating, or affect the digestive function. Studies of yoga, however, have found that with practice, people can learn to consciously decrease their blood pressure, slow the heart rate, reduce the oxygen consumption, alter the circulation, and lower the stress hormone levels. Learning to influence these automatic functions is a different set of skills from those we use to ride a bicycle or kick a soccer ball. Learning to regulate your breath is the first step in discovering how to influence other essential involuntary bodily functions.

Left on its own, breathing does not require your conscious attention to consume oxygen or eliminate carbon dioxide. This is a good thing. Day and night, respiratory centres deep in your brain stem monitor levels of gases in your body and automatically adjust your breathing rate and depth of breathing. As anyone with asthma can tell you, having to pay attention to breathing, in order to get enough life-sustaining oxygen into your body, is not desirable. Every human being is capable of temporarily overriding autonomic control of breathing, by speeding up, slowing down, or holding the breath.

Conscious alteration of the usually automatic breathing process has powerful effects on your mind and body, and it provides a window into your ability to influence other autonomic functions. While you have your attention on your breath, you can modify it, whereas as soon as you relinquish conscious control, your involuntary nervous system resumes its authority. Learning the techniques offered by a pranayama practice will help you to use your breath to influence your physical and mental states, allowing you to create higher states of awareness, adding to a higher quality of life.

Difficulty Breathing?

Ineffective breathing is shallow or laboured and prevents your body from getting the oxygen it needs. Like other symptoms, it can have several causes.

Causes of Breathing Problems

When an area of the body hurts, the natural response is to tense the muscles in that area. This is so automatic that you're often unaware of how much tension you are carrying. Muscle tension can change how you move. It may make you move more slowly, or your posture may change so that your chest is not as open, leaving less room for your lungs to expand effectively. Shallow breathing may cause muscles to become weak and deconditioned. And this does not only affect your breathing muscles; the core muscles of your abdomen and the small muscles of your back can also be affected. When muscles become deconditioned, they are less efficient and require more energy and oxygen to perform activities.

Excess weight can also cause shortness of breath. Additional weight increases the amount of energy you use and therefore the amount of oxygen you need. Weight also increases the workload for the heart. If excess weight is combined with restricted movement and poor posture, your body will struggle to get the oxygen it needs. Certain chronic pain conditions can directly impact posture and contribute to reduced lung capacity. The list may include scoliosis and osteoporosis, which are severe forms of arthritis that cause a degeneration of the bones in the neck and back. Other causes of breathing problems include chronic lung diseases such as emphysema, chronic bronchitis, and asthma. These conditions usually require special medication and sometimes supplemental oxygen in addition to self-management techniques.

Struggling to breathe can be frightening, and this fear can cause two additional problems. First, when you're afraid, you release hormones such as epinephrine, and this can create a vicious cycle of more muscle tension and more shortness of breath. Out of fear that it will hurt you, you may stop activity altogether. If this happens, you cannot build up the endurance necessary to help manage your chronic pain.

Prepare Your Life for Your Breathwork

As with yoga postures, Asana, the number one condition for pranayama practice is to respect your limits. All beginners should start slowly with a few repetitions of simple pranayama techniques, under the guidance of a teacher. As with all yoga practices, pranayama should be increased slowly and regularly. The rate of increase may depend on age, gender, life situation, availability of help, and the ability to contain and channel prana. For example, if you're a former smoker, you may have to take this powerful detoxification slowly, with short, regular rounds. Doing too many rounds will usually lead to lightheadedness and dizziness and can overheat the system. If you notice the signs, respect your body's messages and rest in a seated position or in child's pose. Resume your practice the following day with slightly fewer repetitions, continuing in this way until you feel you are ready to explore a gentle lengthening of your practice. Beginners should always start with abdominal breath and then progress to the full yogic breath.

Set up your body, mind, and space for a pranayama practice:

• Set up your space! Make sure you have a comfortable yoga mat or cushions. It is also important to be in a well-ventilated space. You can consider recharging your space with essential oils or incense. If you are considering essential oils, you can choose them according to your dosha. Scents like eucalyptus oil, rose oil, and holy basil could make your breathing easier and improve your energy.

- Sound vibrations are powerful. You can add soft background music or use a mantra.
- Start with a clean physical body. Clear out your nasal passages. You may use a Neti pot if you wish; this helps clear blockages. It's really important to clear the passages as mucus causes many blockages in the system.
- Ideally, a pranayama practice should be done in the morning before breakfast, but if you can't make it in the morning, then make some time in this day for this powerful practice.
- Get assistance! Forming new habits can be hard, and this breathwork requires consistency. Make sure you have someone there that you can call on when you need some extra guidance. At the very least, ask someone to keep you accountable. Share your goals with them and have them keep you on task.

The practice of pranayama is directly involved with awakening, expanding, and directing prana, the life force energy of the human body, your inner creative force. These are not just breathing exercises.

Breathwork Exercises

Just as there are many causes of ineffective breathing, there are many things you can do to manage this problem. When you feel short of breath, don't stop what you were doing or hurry to finish the task. Instead, slow down. If shortness of breath continues, stop for a few minutes. If your doctor prescribes medication for this problem, then take it. The basic rule is to take things slowly and gradually.

In this next section, I will share with you several tools that can help you achieve better, more effective breathing. Like the other teachings you'll find in this book, understanding and exercising breath is another way to fine-tune the body, as the instrument that it is. These breathing techniques will help you cultivate a stronger connection to your breathing, better manage stress, improve lung capacity, and boost overall well-being. I believe that learning how to use your breath effectively is instrumental in managing your chronic pain.

Abdominal Breathing

The first pranayama technique that students of yoga should master is abdominal breathing. This fundamental technique forms the basis of many pranayama techniques, so it must be mastered over a few days before you attempt any others. It's a simple technique that has powerful effects if done on a regular basis.

Benefits

Abdominal breathing tunes into the functioning of your lungs, calms your physiology, and helps relieve stress and anger. It stabilizes your emotions and balances your hormones. It also improves your sleep quality and helps trigger the relaxation response in your physiology. And with each deep inhalation and exhalation, you are oxygenating, circulating, rejuvenating, and detoxifying in an efficient way.

Technique

The best way to begin this technique is to lie flat on your back with your hands over your belly button, forming a diamond shape. Do this by touching your right and left thumb above your bellybutton, and your right and left index finger below your belly button.

Begin by exhaling fully and squeezing the abdomen gently backwards toward the spine. As you release the abdomen it will naturally rise with the next inhalation. Take it slowly! Complete long inhalations before moving to extra slow exhalations.

117

Elbows should be fully rested. If your abdominal muscles feel tight, it can be helpful to practice in a supine position with a bolster beneath the knees, if you have tight hamstrings or low back pain. For optimal results, practice for 5 to 10 minutes.

Full Yogic Breath

The second pranayama technique that students of yoga should master is full yogic breathing, sometimes called a three-part yogic breath. The fundamental technique forms the basis of pranayama techniques, so it must be mastered over a few days before you attempt other techniques. Three-part breath can be done while you are lying on your back with one hand on the chest and one hand on the abdomen, or in the seated cross-legged position. The breath is taken in and expelled in three parts to ensure the full use of lung capacity.

Benefits
The benefits are the same as abdominal breathing; however, this breath technique has more energizing benefits.

Technique
First, exhale completely. In order to inhale, the diaphragm drops in, and the abdomen expands, drawing the breath into the lower lungs. Next, the ribs expand laterally, filling the middle of the lungs. Finally, the clavicle rises up as breath continues to be drawn into the upper lungs.

You may notice that your abdomen sinks slightly as your chest expands. This is natural, however, as you may be in the habit of clavicular breathing. When this happens, continue the focus on the abdomen and the first part of the full yogic breath in order to counteract the tendency to breathe mostly in the upper lungs. On the exhalation, the diaphragm relaxes, causing the clavicle to sink; the rib cage contracts, and finally the body sinks backwards toward the spine. Return to the natural rhythm of your breath. Observe the effects of this pranayama on your body, energy, breath, and mind. For optimal results, practice for 5 to 10 minutes.

Purification Breath (Kapalabathi)

The next breathing technique in Sanskrit is Kapalabathi, which translates as "shining skull purification exercise." This exercise sends the breath to the frontal lobe of the brain, activating and energizing this area to help bring shining clarity to one's thoughts. It is an invigorating technique that uses dynamic exhalation to expel toxins and unnecessary emotions that accumulate in the frontal lobe. It also helps move mucus out of the sinus passages, so it is good to have some tissues nearby. You should only attempt this once you're comfortable with abdominal breathing, as Kapalabathi requires a sensitive understanding of the lungs, and relative looseness and flexibility in the abdominal muscles.

Benefits

Purification breath has great benefits for immunity, blood purification, allergies, and sinus problems. It is also good for toning the abdominal muscles and improving digestion. You should not practice this technique if you have high blood pressure, a headache, or bad constipation. It is not advisable for women who are pregnant or on their menstrual cycle.

More benefits are:

- Detoxification of the frontal lobe of the brain.
- Purification of the respiratory system by reducing phlegm.
- Strengthening of the immune system.

- Relief of asthma and sinus problems.
  Improvement in the expulsion of carbon dioxide and absorption of oxygen.
- Purification of the blood.
- Toning of the digestive system and abdominal muscles.
- Improvement in skin health.

Technique

This exercise is performed in a seated position with the spine upright and the eyes closed.

- Place your hands on your knees and connect your thumbs and index fingers.
- Close your eyes or soften your gaze and send your attention to the middle of your forehead.
- Relax your face, relax your eyebrows and shoulders, and retain a subtle smile on your face.
- Take a long, relaxed breath out, and inhale that exhale through the nose by drawing the navel in toward the spine.
- Dynamically exhale and allow the inhale to occur naturally.
- Continue the cycle of dynamic exhales for at least 30 rounds to begin with.
- At the end, completely exhale and apply the root lock by gently lifting the pelvic floor upward very gently. Hold the breath out to your capacity, for approximately 5 to 10 seconds.
- Then while maintaining the root lock, take a deep inhale. At the top of the inhale, retain the breath and apply a throat lock by dropping the chin to the chest, and almost imagine you're swallowing. Hold this breath in, according to your capacity, for approximately 5 to10 seconds.
- Release the throat lock, lift up your chin, and slowly exhale. Take three full yogic breaths and observe the flow of prana. Your breath cycles should be long, slow, smooth, and happy.

Alternate Nostril Breathing

The next technique is called alternate nostril breathing or Anuloma Viloma pranayama. This gentle technique has powerful healing capabilities. It balances the active and passive energies of the body's solar and lunar channels, which is said to flow through our right and left nostrils, respectively. Solar energy is the energy of getting things done. Lunar energy is our compassion, receptivity, and intuitive power.

When you are overly solar influenced, you become forceful, aggressive, and hot. When you are overly lunar influenced, you become too passive, dispassionate, and unproductive. By balancing both energies, we can better leverage each of them.

Benefits

Alternate nostril breathing cools the system, creating a sense of calm and peace, while simultaneously energizing us, boosting our immune system, and purifying the blood. It quickly tackles the usual culprits of stress, dissolving anxiety from the mind. It also improves concentration and focus. Research has shown that alternate nostril breathing has an immediate effect on the toning of the parasympathetic nervous system and the calming of the entire physiology.

Technique

Alternate nostril breathing can be practiced on the floor or in a chair.

- Sit upright with your spine straight and your shoulders relaxed.
- Hold your head upright.
- Hold your right hand up with fingers extended.
- Straighten your little finger and ring finger and thumb.
- Touch your left thumb to left index finger resting it upward on the left knee.

- Close your eyes and take one full inhale and exhale as you would in full yogic breathing.
- After the exhale, close your right nostril, using the pad of your thumb, and inhale gently into the left nostril, all the way down to the belly.
- Hold your breath in for a moment and close the left nostril with your right index finger and little finger. Then release from the right nostril and exhale completely through your right nostril.
- From the bottom of your lungs, hold the emptiness for a moment; then inhale through the right nostril, all the way down to the belly.
- Hold your breath for a moment, and then open the left nostril, close the right nostril, and exhale completely from the belly up, out of the left nostril. This completes one round.

Throughout, take care that your breathing is silent and your body is still. Take time with your inhales and exhales—6 to 8 seconds—and hold your breath for 1 to 2 seconds.

Always begin this practice with one full yogic breath; then inhale through the left nostril, exhale right, inhale right, and end with an exhale to the left nostril. About 7 to 10 rounds of the sequence will offer great benefits for everyone, but especially for those who want to overcome an overly reactive nature. You can increase the rounds up to 20 over a few weeks if you are seeking deeper benefits.

Remember this:

- Breathe joy into each day.
- Breathe clarity into each moment.
- Breathe through your pain.
- Breathe positivity into your perspective.
- Breathe health into all your cells.
- Breathe!

Chapter 7

Understanding Your Negative Emotions

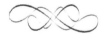

"Do not resist the pain. Allow it to be there.
Surrender to the grief, despair, fear, loneliness,
or whatever form the suffering takes.
Witness it without labeling it mentally.
Allow it to be there. Embrace it.

Then see the miracle of surrendering.
Transmuting deep suffering into deep peace."

Eckhart Tolle

Your thoughts have power. Regardless of where you are in the world, you will always be in your own head. When you live each day with chronic pain, it may create negative emotions. You feel angry—at the world, at others for not understanding what you are feeling, at your own body, and at yourself. Chronic pain can turn your thoughts on you, making your everyday world a dark place to live. This can create a vicious cycle where your pain becomes stronger and you then give it even more strength with the power of your negative emotions.

A chronic condition resulting in chronic pain can be accompanied by a host of other symptoms.

These symptoms are an indication that your body mechanisms are in a state of imbalance. Therefore, understanding how to manage these symptoms effectively can help you directly influence your experience of pain and make you a better self-manager. When you take control over your own pain management, it gives you a sense of power, which can then help you also manage your negative thoughts effectively, removing you from the vicious cycle that is giving strength to your pain.

One of the benefits to taking control of your emotions is that it allows you to understand your pain from a place of calm knowledge and make decisions from this place. It takes you out of a place where you are making irrational emotional responses, and into a place where you can rationally move forward to greater healing. It allows you to begin to be able to communicate what your experience of living with chronic pain is, to yourself and those who love you.

I understand how difficult it is to experience these symptoms and not be able to effectively communicate what you are feeling to those around you.

When you have a better understanding and acceptance of what you are experiencing beyond just your pain, you can become not only an effective self-manager but also an effective communicator and can self-advocate to friends, family, and healthcare professionals.

Here are some common symptoms that lead to the negative thought/pain cycle, and some self-management tools:

- Fatigue
- Fear
- Sleep problems
- Depression
- Anger

Fatigue

Unfortunately, fatigue is often misunderstood by those who do not live with chronic pain. After all, others don't see or experience your fatigue. Spouses, family members, and friends sometimes do not understand the unpredictable way in which the fatigue associated with your condition can affect you. They may think that you are just not interested in certain activities or that you want to be alone.

Chronic pain can drain your energy, making fatigue a very real problem. It is not just your pain that prevents you from doing the things you love, but also your fatigue. Sometimes you may not even know why you feel so tired. To manage fatigue, it is important for you to understand that your fatigue may be related to several factors, including the following:

- **Less efficient use of energy** – Chronic pain or other chronic conditions cause the body to use energy less efficiently. This is because energy that could be consumed for everyday activities are instead being redirected to the parts of your body affected by your condition. Therefore, your brain may release chemical signals to conserve energy and make you rest more.

- **Lack of movement** – Muscles that are not used regularly, become weak very quickly and are less efficient at doing what they are supposed to do. This can happen to all the muscles in your body, including the heart, which is made of muscle tissue. When the heart becomes deconditioned, its ability to pump blood decreases. Your blood carries necessary nutrients and oxygen to other parts of the body. When muscles do not receive these nutrients and oxygen, they cannot function properly. Deconditioned muscles exhaust more easily than muscles in good condition. Less muscle means less strength and less energy... a vicious cycle being created that can result in fatigue. Are you moving within your tolerance?

- **Poor nourishment** – Food is your basic source of energy. If you eat low quality food, eat too much or too little, or improperly digest food, this can result in fatigue. Your path to feeling well begins in your kitchen. Are you eating healthy, whole foods?

- **Inadequate rest** – People with chronic pain either overdo or underdo activity, and some do not balance activity with rest. Learning pacing, as discussed in an earlier chapter, is key to you becoming an effective self-manager. Are you pacing activities with the rest periods, and are you getting enough good quality sleep?

- **Negative emotions** – Emotions such as anxiety/worry, fear, boredom, and depression can cause fatigue. It can be exhausting to deal with the ongoing stressors that can accompany chronic pain. Most people are aware of the connection between stress and feeling tired, but are you aware that fatigue may be a major symptom of depression? Are you effectively managing stress?

- **Medication** – Some medications, including those you are taking for your pain, can cause fatigue. If you think your fatigue is related to your medication, talk to your doctor. Sometimes medication or dosages can be changed. If fatigue is a problem, start by trying to determine the cause. Again, a journal may be helpful.

Consider that some of these causes of fatigue are within your control to improve and change. If you answered no to any of the above questions, you may have found one or more of the reasons for your fatigue. The important thing to remember is that your fatigue may be caused by things other than your pain. Therefore, to combat and prevent fatigue, you must address all the possible causes. This may mean trying a variety of self-management tools.

Practice to Overcome Fatigue

Practice suggestions:

Pick one area of your life; for example, your physical health. For a week, make new choices in the moment that support future health. This could be eating whole grains, going to bed earlier, avoiding watching the news right before bedtime, taking a morning walk, or a combination of choices. At the end of the week, notice how you feel, physically and emotionally. Appreciate yourself for your new choices.

If you practice an exercise routine or yoga poses, pick one that you can do fairly easily. Without harming yourself, hold this pose for twice as long as you normally would. Notice your inner dialogue when the pose becomes uncomfortable. Do you blame the pose, or yourself, for your suffering? Do you want out? Consider that perhaps your fatigue comes from your attitude and not from the sensations themselves.

The next time you're upset, notice your physiological responses, such as increased tension in your muscles, changes in your breath, or tightness in your belly. How much time during the day do you spend in this state? Is this the way you want to spend your life? Choose to let go of suffering in this very moment.

Create your own intention for daily living. Write it out. Read it again when you need to. Write it out again when you need to. It can be something like:

- I can release all suffering and live life right now.
- Life may be difficult, but I do not need to suffer.

Fear

"Nothing in life is to be feared; it is only to be understood.
Now is the time to understand more, so that we may fear less."
– Marie Curie

Fear generally is a common problem for us all, and especially for my clients facing chronic pain.

We all have some measure of fear every day. Understand that the fear you experience could be of short duration or a long-lasting fear. When a fear is long-lasting and persistent, this may be experienced as anxiety or panic.

Another aspect of fear is anger, which is actually an attempt to defend against a threat that you perceive is coming. One of the most interesting things about fear is that it exists in relationship to the future. Consider this if you are actually involved in a situation that needs you to fight for your life and there is no time to be afraid. The sympathetic nervous system is mobilizing for you to run, and your body functions are operating on full blast. Your nervous system is not distracted by thinking in the abstract about what may happen in the future; rather, it is dealing with what is happening in the moment. It is only when you think about what might happen or what could've happened that you feel afraid. Is it possible to live without fear? Yes, with improved awareness of what causes your fear, you can become better at managing it.

Choose to observe your fears on a daily basis, and continually bring awareness back to what is happening in the present moment.

Practice to Overcome Fear

Try this version of a basic relaxation pose:

- Gather together two blankets, a cloth the size of a face towel, and a pillow. Find a quiet place and sit down on the floor.
- Fold one blanket into a large rectangle and then roll it. Place the blanket roll under your knees and cover your feet and legs with the other blanket.
- Using your elbows for support, slowly lie back. Put the pillow under your head.
- Bring the blanket up to cover your torso, and place the cloth over your eyes.
- Finally, tuck your arms under the blanket, palms up.
- Your torso and arms should be supported by the floor, and your legs resting completely on the blanket roll.
- Take several long, slow breaths.
- All you have to do right now is to be where you are, doing what you were doing. You do not have to solve any problems or make any demands on yourself.
- Release even more into the support of the floor and the blanket roll, with your limbs heavy, your breath slowing, and your jaw becoming slack.
- Live in this position for 5 to 15 minutes.
- Come out of basic relaxation pose by slowly bending one knee to your chest and rolling to lie on one side. Take a couple of breaths before you use your arms to help you to come to a sitting position. As you gradually stand up, tell yourself that this feeling of relaxation is always available to you. Smile.

Other practice suggestions:

If you are in a situation in which you cannot practice basic relaxation pose, try this exercise. Become aware of being afraid or anxious; bring your attention to those places in your body where you feel sensations. For many of us, that may be in the throat, the diaphragm, or the stomach. Breathe easily, feeling what arises, without judgement or analysis. As you continue to breathe, say out loud to yourself or to a trusted friend, "I am feeling afraid." Your willingness to admit that you are afraid can greatly lessen fear's grip on you.

Regarding the event that is actually causing you fear, put yourself in the situation and then ask yourself what is the worst that can happen? Then ask yourself what would happen. Ask several times. You will notice, and it will become apparent very soon that nothing would be happening. This technique has helped so many of my clients face fear and put it into perspective.

When you acknowledge fear, fear no longer controls you. Acknowledge it and feel it, and in your mind live through your worst fear, and follow it with these helpful hints:

- And then what would happen?
- Right here, right now, I am safe.
- I choose the life that I have right now.
- I am willing to act in the face of fear.
- I can do this.

Sleep

Just like food and water, sleep is a basic human need. Sleep is so important. I talk about this a lot. The reason I talk about it so much is because it can be hard to change our habits before bed, but getting a good night's sleep is key to managing both your pain and your negative thoughts.

Not getting enough sleep can have physiological effects on your body, which makes it even more difficult for you to participate in your daily life. You feel stiff. Your pain feels stronger. Your body feels lethargic.

When you don't get enough sleep, you will have a hard time focusing. You'll find that your mind wanders. It will also be much easier to slip into negative thoughts or emotional responses. Your defenses are down, so you may react to things quickly without rational thought. Lack of sleep can lead to irritability and can strain your relationships with your loved ones.

Practice to Overcome Sleeplessness

There are many ways to help yourself get a better night's sleep. We have talked about this already, so I won't go back into it, other than to share with you this reminder:

- Don't drink or eat right before bed, especially anything with caffeine.
- Turn off your devices and your TV at least an hour before you try to sleep.
- Make sure your bed is comfortable.
- Keep your bedroom at a cooler temperature.

Depression

"Research has shown that chronic pain can be linked to an imbalance of certain neurotransmitters such as serotonin and norepinephrine, causing depression and sleep disorders in chronic pain."
— IAWP

This is such a big topic, I hesitate to address it here, but it does need to be mentioned. I have seen many of my clients go through depression as a result of their chronic pain. The most important thing you need to hear right now, if you think are depressed, is that you need to seek medical help. You may think you can get through this alone, but please don't try. Sometimes your body is so out of balance that you need medication. Don't misunderstand me; I don't think that medication is always the answer, but sometimes it is necessary.

One of the most important things you can do for yourself is to recognize when you are experiencing times of sadness and when you are depressed.

What is depression?

According to the Mayo Clinic, depression is defined in the following way: "Depression is a mood disorder that causes a persistent feeling of sadness and loss of interest. Also called major depressive disorder or clinical depression, it affects how you feel, think, and behave, and can lead to a variety of emotional and physical problems. You may have trouble doing normal day-to-day activities, and sometimes you may feel as if life isn't worth living."[4]

How do you know if you are depressed?

Here is a quick exercise to help you decide if you are experiencing a bout of sadness or depression. Ask yourself the following questions:

- Do I experience pleasure in doing things that I normally love?
- Am I interested in participating in daily life?
- Am I feeling down or hopeless for a long period of time?
- Do I have very little energy throughout the day?
- Do I feel restless?
- Do I have a hard time concentrating?
- Do I wish myself harm or worse?
- Do I have problems falling or staying asleep, or do I sleep too much?
- Do I have a poor appetite or am I overeating?

---

4 https://www.mayoclinic.org/diseases-conditions/depression/symptoms-causes/syc-20356007

If you answered yes to all of these questions, then put the book down and contact your doctor. Otherwise, if you answered yes to 5 or more questions, also contact your doctor to see which treatment options are best for you.

Anger

One of the most common responses to living with chronic pain is anger. You are not alone. Each day, you are met with uncertainty. How will your pain feel today? How will it affect your mood? Will you be able to get your work done? Will it stop you from feeling joy, excitement, or happiness?

Anger is normal. Chronic pain is a challenge, and it is one that is ongoing. That said, your anger can get in the way of your ability to manage your pain. Anger leads you to make irrational decisions. It can lead you to lash out at your loved ones or the people who are trying to help. If you allow your anger to regularly control your response to your chronic pain, you will only make that pain worse.

Yes, allow yourself to feel the anger, but also allow yourself to let it go. Don't beat yourself up for being angry; arm yourself with the tools you need to pull yourself out of anger.

Practice to Overcome Anger

Here are a few practices to help you overcome your anger:

- Cool off! – Allow yourself to recognize your anger. Remove yourself from the situation that is triggering you. If it is your own thoughts, do something to pull yourself from those thoughts. Do something that you really enjoy. Go for a walk to your favourite shop. Make yourself a tea. Read a few pages of an engaging book.
- Journal – Write about your anger as a way of releasing it. Make a promise to yourself that once the words hit the page, you will do your best to let

134

that anger go. The next time you find that same trigger causing you to feel angry again, remind yourself that you are bigger than the negative feelings it is creating. You are stronger.

- Ask yourself if you are justified in being angry. Sometimes the thing that is making you angry is worth being angry at.

You Are Strong

Sadness, depression, fear, and lack of sleep are only some of the symptoms you may be facing that are causing negative emotions to take control of your everyday life and get in the way of you managing your pain. Daily life can be stressful, and these symptoms can also cause things like memory problems and even job loss. These things feel big. They are challenges that if you let them, they can take control of your life. These challenges will stop you from becoming the effective self-manager I know you can be.

You are always stronger than you think. You have so many tools you can use to help pull yourself out of the darker moments. Remember, you don't have to do it alone. Reach out for help, especially if you feel you are depressed.

Calming Meditation

To end this chapter, I'd like to share a calming meditation with you to help you in those moments when you need help managing your negative emotions:

Alternate nostril breathing (Anuloma Viloma)

This practice of alternating between the right and left nostrils as you inhale and exhale, unblocks and purifies the nadis, the "energy passages that carry life force and cosmic energy through the body."

Studies show that seven days of practicing this technique rebalances an overactive nervous system. And a study of 90 people with high blood pressure found that alternate nostril breathing lowered blood pressure and improved mental focus.

Instructions:

- Take a comfortable seated position.
- Close your right hand and release the thumb, the ring finger, and the little finger.
- Gently close your right nostril with your thumb.
- Inhale through your left nostril; then close it with your ring finger.
- Open your right nostril and exhale slowly through it. Inhale through the right nostril then close it. Open your left nostril and exhale slowly through it that completes one cycle.
- Repeat 3 to 5 times.

Once completed, rest your attention on the center of your forehead and notice any bodily sensations. Move this attention to the top of your crown. If you feel your mind wavering, come back to your breath and focus on the exhale. Try to hold this meditation, starting with about two minutes and slowly progressing over time to 20 minutes.

Chapter 8

Communicate Your Needs
to Your Healthcare Professionals

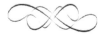

*"The single biggest problem in communication is
the illusion that it has taken place.*
– George Bernard Shaw

8

Communication is a necessity at all times, but especially when you are communicating things that are important to you, and especially when managing a long-term condition. When you are managing chronic pain and the symptoms of chronic pain, good communication becomes your lifeline. It is the key to becoming the best self-manager you can be. Understanding how to communicate your needs to your healthcare provider will also help you develop healthy coping skills.

You have to become a strong self-advocate. This means really understanding your condition and how it affects you personally. In doing so, you represent yourself effectively and your healthcare team can understand you.

I understand that advice and recommendations from your doctors and other healthcare professionals can be confusing at times; therefore, knowing that you may ask questions empowers you to prevent any further problems from arising.

From my own involvement in the healthcare system, personally and professionally, I understand how sometimes my clients are afraid to talk freely, or they feel there's not enough time during an appointment. You may not want to share personal and possibly embarrassing information, and healthcare professionals may use words that you do not understand.

Stop now and consider what challenges you may be experiencing that hinder your communication with your healthcare providers. To find your blocks to open and honest communication, answer these questions:

1. Do I feel embarrassed to talk about some of the things that are happening with me physically or even emotionally?

2. If the answer to question #1 is *yes,* ask yourself: Why am I embarrassed? I know this can be a tough one to define, but be as honest with yourself as you can.
3. Do you know how to talk clearly about what you are feeling?
4. What words do you use to describe your pain?
5. Do you feel like there is enough time in your appointments to talk with your healthcare providers?
6. What don't you understand about your pain? It could be things like what makes it worse or why you are experiencing some of the symptoms that you are.
7. Is your fear or anxiety hindering your communication with your providers? If so, what are you afraid of?
8. Do you understand your medications—when to take them and why you are taking them?

Once you've answered these questions, take some time to reflect on your answers. Can you see how developing your ability to communicate what your chronic pain feels like, and how it is affecting your body, can help you self-manage your care?

In this chapter, I am going to help you communicate your needs with your healthcare providers be giving you a few easy tools to work with. In the next chapter, I will address the importance of communicating with your loved ones.

Get in the Driver's Seat!

Many of us would like our healthcare providers to be like warm-hearted computers. We want their brains to know everything about the human body so that they can tell us exactly what is happening with our own individual bodies. We want our doctors, therapists, and specialists to be able to make the perfect diagnosis all the time, prescribe the perfect medication that will yield immediate results, and come up with a treatment plan that will effectively manage the pain. We also expect that they will be empathetic and caring, making us feel that we are their only patient. Basically, we want them to be superheroes.

I can tell you, after decades of experience as a therapist within the Canadian healthcare system, I care about each and every patient. Does that mean that I am able to behave in the way I just described in the last paragraph, with every patient in every meeting? Of course not! I do my very best as a healthcare provider to understand your pain and address it, but I can only do so much. As you know already, chronic pain is complicated. While you may have a similar diagnosis to many of my other patients, it doesn't mean that I am able to read your mind and understand what you are feeling personally. You are an individual with individual physical, emotional, and spiritual needs. As we also discussed, all of these levels of who you are and how you exist in this world have an impact on your chronic pain.

Healthcare providers may sometimes come across as being poor communicators, which may feel intimidating to you. They may come across as too busy to take the time to talk, or you may feel that they are not taking the time to understand your specific concerns. Often, the system is stretched and they are busy, but always remember that they are and should be there for you. Although you do not have to become best friends with your healthcare providers, you should expect them to be attentive and caring.

Also understand that your healthcare providers, especially when it comes to chronic pain, may not have all the answers. It is important to note that with something like chronic pain that has physical, mental, emotional, and spiritual manifestations, there is not one sole provider that can provide you all the answers. The approach is for you to have a **team** behind you to support different aspects toward your well-being. Think of it as an umbrella of care, with each contributing a step toward your road to well-being. A relationship with your healthcare providers is much like a business partnership or even a marriage. Establishing and maintaining this long-term relationship may take some effort, but it can make a large difference to your health. You need to be in the driver's seat to understand your condition. You need to be able to communicate to be your best representative.

The bottom line: Healthcare providers have devoted their lives to the work they do because they care about the people they serve, but they do need help from you so that they can give you the individualized care you need. If you want to have the most positive impact from your interactions with your healthcare providers, you have to get in the driver's seat.

ACT

"The way we communicate with others and with ourselves ultimately determines the quality of our lives."
– Tony Robbins

You might be thinking that you have tried to get in the driver's seat. You might be thinking: "Sure, sure, Theven, that is easier said than done." What I've shared with you about you having to take more control of your interactions in the healthcare system through clearer communication, may even make you angry. Or you may be feeling very overwhelmed in this moment.

I understand. But know that once you learn how to take a more active role in your health care, you will ultimately become healthier, happier, and in control of your pain. Why? Because you will be able to ask for exactly the kind of individualized care you need. Keep in mind as I say this, that the work is ongoing. It will never be a perfect process, but it will always be one that you can manage in the end.

The best way to receive the care you need from your healthcare providers is to ACT.

A - Anticipate

C - Communicate

T - Take action

Anticipate

When you live with chronic pain, you are often dealing with multiple healthcare providers because one provider will not have all of the answers. You are probably already doing this, so you know how confusing and often frustrating this can be. Sometimes this means that you will have multiple appointments with people who don't understand your pain history. While you may wish that you could walk into every appointment and the person you are meeting with would already understand what you are going through and how they can help you, it's just not possible.

Begin by creating a calendar, listing all your appointments. Include the healthcare provider's name and what they do. You might be meeting with your family doctor, pain specialist, physiotherapist, nutritionist, psychologist, or social worker, to name a few. Prior to going to your meeting, the best thing you can do is anticipate this reality and prepare yourself for the appointment. How can you do this? By understanding your pain, knowing what you need, and being able to clearly describe your pain.

Once you have your schedule of appointments mapped out, ask yourself if you understand what each practitioner does and how they can help you. For example, many people are often confused about the role of social workers. They do very important work, often in the areas of connecting you to life-changing educational and health-related resources. If you are feeling isolated in your home, they can help you find a community centre with social programs. If you are having a difficult time communicating with your loved ones about your condition, they can facilitate a meeting with you to get you started. If you don't know why your doctor has referred you to someone, you can reach out to them and ask.

The next step is to create an appointment agenda. Ask yourself what you want to achieve in the appointment. Write out a series of questions that you have for the specialist you are meeting. Sometimes it can be hard to know what to ask right away. Remember that there are no stupid questions. Start by making a question out of your goal. Let's take the example I used with the social worker. Maybe your goal is to meet other people who have a similar condition to yours.

Goal
- I want to meet other people with fibromyalgia.

Questions for your social worker:
- Are there any social groups for people with fibromyalgia?
- Are there any exercise groups or classes, like yoga for people with fibromyalgia or chronic pain?
- Does my healthcare plan cover any of the costs of attending these groups?
- What is the process to apply to attend one of these groups?
- I will have a hard time finding a ride; can I apply for transportation?

Take some time to really think about what you want and how each healthcare provider might be able to help you. Don't worry if you think you might be asking the wrong person. Often, they can direct you to the right person!

Your Pain Profile

The next steps will help you to clearly communicate what your pain feels like and how it affects your daily life in all areas: physical, emotional, social, and spiritual.

Preparing your pain profile:

When did the pain start?

_____

Was there a specific cause (e.g., a fall) or did it just seem to develop over time?

_____

Has it gotten worse with time, or has it remained the same?

_____

Is it intermittent or constant?

_____

Does it come in waves and then subside? Yes □ No □

What does the pain feel like? (Refer to Figure (table above) on page (#))

Flickering	Drilling	Grueling
Quivering	Stabbing	Vicious
Pulsing	Sharp	Killing
Throbbing	Cutting	Terrifying
Beating	Hot	Intense
Pounding	Dull	Unbearable
Jumping	Sore	Fearful
Flashing	Itching	Tearing
Shooting	Hot	Cool
Pricking	Sickening	Nagging
Boring	Suffocating	Nauseating

_____

Is there a time of day when the pain is worse?

_____

Does it wake you from sleep? Yes ☐ No ☐

Does it cause insomnia? Yes ☐ No ☐

Have you ever had this type of pain before? Yes ☐ No ☐

When?

_____

Why?

_____

What increases the pain? Sitting? _____ Lying down? _____ Mild massage? _____

Other?

_____

Does the pain radiate to another part of your body such as your back or legs? Yes ☐ No ☐

How severe is your pain? On a scale from 0 to 10, with 10 being the most severe, how does this pain rate? 0 1 2 3 4 5 6 7 8 9 10

Can you distract yourself from the pain either partially or completely? Or is the pain so intense that distraction is impossible?

_____

How does it affect the quality of your life? Have you stopped visiting friends? Are you irritable, angry, depressed?

_____

Is the pain accompanied by symptoms such as nausea, sweating, or shortness of breath?

_____

Which, if any, medications have you taken?

_____

_____

Have they relieved the pain?
Completely? Yes □ No □
Partially? Yes □ No □
Not at all? Yes □ No □

Are you sensitive or allergic to any pain medication?

_____

Miscellaneous comments:

_____

_____

_____

Use Your Words!

Prior to going to your appointment, write out some of the words you can use to describe your pain. Here is a list to get you started:

These words were developed in 1970 by Dr. Malzak, and used in the McGill Pain Questionnaire. You can find the full list here: *Living a Healthy life with Chronic Pain* by Lefort, Lorig, Sobel, Gonzalez

Here are a few examples of ways you can use some of these words:

- The pain in the back of my skull is **nauseating**.
- It feels like someone is **drilling** behind my eyes.
- The pain in my back **radiates** down my leg.
- My muscles feel **tender** to the touch.
- My knees are **aching**.
- I have a **shooting** pain in shoulder.
- There is a **dull** ache in my lower back that never goes away.

The more descriptive you can get when talking about your pain to your healthcare providers, the better they will understand what you are going through and be able to help you. Take a moment now to write out some sentences, like the ones I have above, for your pain.

The next layer of information you can give your healthcare providers is to rate the level of your pain.

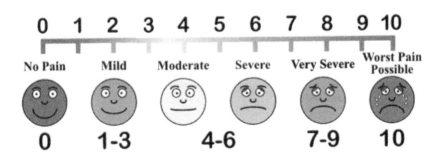

This is not an exact science, and that doesn't matter. The more information you can share, the more appropriate your care will be. Try now to take the sentences you wrote and add a pain rating next to it. I'll do the same with the sentences I've create above to give you an example. I've also added further description to help you see how I've come up with the number.

- The pain in the back of my skull is **nauseating**. (9 – The pain makes me want to stay in bed because I feel so sick.)
- It feels like someone is **drilling** behind my eyes. (8 – I can go about my daily activities but there are moments when the pain takes over.)
- The pain in my back **radiates** down my leg. (10 – When it radiates, I can't move.)
- My muscles feel **tender** to the touch. (4 – If I don't touch the muscle, I don't feel the pain as much. The pain is annoying, but it doesn't hinder my daily life.)
- My knees are **aching**. (6 – The discomfort can make me feel depressed because I am worried it will get worse.)
- I have a **shooting** pain in my shoulder. (7 – It really hurts to move my arm, so I often make a choice to use my other hand.)
- There is a **dull** ache in my lower back that never goes away. (3 – It's uncomfortable to sit in the same position at times.)

Don't get too stuck on getting the exact number. Also, know that the number you assign can not only change daily but throughout a single day.

To sum up this section on anticipating your appointments so that you can get the most out of them, follow these 3 easy steps:

1. Create an appointment agenda. Know who you are going to see, why you are going to see them, and how they can help you.
2. Develop a list of questions for the healthcare provider you are meeting with, even if you don't know that they are the person who can answer them.

3. Understand your pain so that you can clearly describe it to your healthcare providers. Create your pain profile, use your words, and rate your pain!

Communicate

Now that you have begun to understand your pain more clearly and how it is affecting your life, you have given yourself some powerful tools to be able to communicate with your healthcare providers. Your ultimate goal is to get the best care available to you.

In your communication:

*   Be clear.
*   Be honest.
*   Be direct.

The only way you can get the help you need is to be open and honest. If the healthcare provider you are meeting with doesn't have all of the information, how can they be expected to provide you with the best possible care? If you feel rushed in an appointment, or like you aren't being heard, find a nice way to let them know.

The best thing to always remember is that doctors, nurses, therapists, and any other specialist you might meet are all people. They don't know you, but they do want to help you. Help them to help you by being open with your needs and your concerns. I know sometimes this can feel very overwhelming. Sometimes you don't even really know what your needs are. This is okay! You are human too.

When you've anticipated these appointments before they happen, you can bring that knowledge with you. Write it down so that you can remind yourself in the moment what you want to say. It's okay to feel nervous, anxious, or even frustrated. This is normal, but do your best to not let it get in the way of your care!

Take Action

Your work is not done once you leave the appointment. Take some time to reflect on how the appointment went. Were you able to clearly communicate how your pain was affecting you, either physically, emotionally, spiritually, or socially, depending on who you were meeting with?

Did you effectively prepare for the appointment? Were your questions answered? Did you feel heard? If you did not feel heard, can you do anything to advocate for yourself in the future?

Remember that your chronic pain needs ongoing management. While you are reflecting on your appointment, ask yourself:

1. When do I follow up with this professional?
2. Should I seek a second opinion?
3. Is there another provider I can reach out to for help? (Especially if you didn't feel your needs were met.)
4. Was I given any homework? (For example, did your physiotherapist give you some simple exercises to do from home? If so, create a schedule to do these exercises and keep on yourself to do them.)

Taking action on what you learn in these appointments is so important. If you don't follow through on your end, all of the work can be wasted. I know it can be overwhelming to navigate the healthcare system, but you can do it. Give yourself the tools you need. Allow yourself the time you need. Know that people do want to help you receive the best care. Advocate for yourself. Take your care into your hands by taking action!

Chapter 9

Nurturing Strong Communication in Relationships

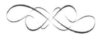

*"Emotional awareness is necessary so you can properly convey
your thoughts and feelings to the other person."*
– Jason Goldberg

Yes, while it's important to live a healthy life, eat well, sleep well, exercise, and have an overall sense of well-being on a physical level, if you don't have a connectedness to all those around you, then you are missing an essential key to well-being.

In South Africa where I grew up, it is said you can have everything, but if you don't have Ubuntu, you have nothing.

Have you heard of Ubuntu? It is an African principle that means "I am because we are." It is all about community. There is a beautiful story about an anthropologist who placed a basket of candy near a tree and asked the children to stand 100 metres away. He told the children that when he said go, they could all race toward the candy, and whoever got there first could have it all.

When the race began, the children joined hands and ran together. When they reached the basket, they shared the candy equally. When the anthropologist asked them why, they replied, "Ubuntu."

You might be wondering why I shared this story to start a chapter on communicating your needs with your family and friends. It is simple: People want to help you. Your loved ones don't want to see you suffering in pain and, I can imagine, in most cases, would do anything to help take that pain away. The same goes for your friends. The people who care about you are a part of your community, and you are a part of theirs.

One of the greatest gifts you can give the ones you love is the opportunity to understand how they can help you, and then to give them that opportunity. I know this can be hard. I know that you might be reading this right now and thinking that you've tried and they can't give you what you need. I am here to help you try again or to try for the first time. Communication is a skill to be developed. When your community knows what you need, they will serve your wellness needs, meeting you where you are and guiding you to where you want to be!

Develop Your Communication Skills

"Be a blessing to others and you will be blessed."
– Proverbs 11:25

When speaking about relationships, I refer to a sense of physical connection to all those around you, with emphasis on your relationship with yourself and your relationship to a sense of community.

Now relationships can bring us joy, but they can also bring us stress. They definitely impact our everyday lives and therefore our health.

Let's take a closer look. Relationships are a big part of our well-being. We have many relationships in our lives, from spouses to partners, to parents, to children, to siblings, to co-workers, to neighbours. We have intimate relationships, social relationships, and professional relationships. Relationships are not something we can escape, because people make up the world. Whether you want to admit it or not, you need people, both on a personal and a professional level. Learning to navigate your relationships in a healthy way can really improve your well-being.

Pain can get in the way of our interaction with others. Your pain can distract you so that you don't listen very well when others are speaking to you. Pain can create a host of emotions, making you feel angry and irritable. These feelings can impact your judgement and may cause you to express these feelings inappropriately to family, friends, and co-workers. Pain may also make you feel overwhelmed, and this may cause you to withdraw. When pain becomes your focus, this creates a problem as your communication becomes centred solely around you and your pain.

You know you care about your close family and friends and other relationships that are important to you, but a breakdown in your communication can result in poor relationships. Often, you may end up feeling that nobody understands you, and this frustration can lead to a feeling of helplessness, isolation, and depression. Such feelings can exacerbate your feeling of chronic pain.

When communication breaks down, it affects your pain and symptoms. Your thoughts can directly affect physical sensations in the body. Your muscles tense, blood sugar and blood pressure levels may rise, and there's increased strain on the heart. Pain may interfere with concentration, which sometimes leads to accidents. Clearly, poor communication is bad for your physical, mental, and emotional health.

To become an effective self-manager of your pain, noticing these cycles and having effective communication skills is essential.

In this chapter, I will discuss tools to improve communication. These tools are intended for you to express your feelings in a positive way. The key is to minimize conflict, learn to ask for support, and know when to say *no*. You will also learn how to apply effective listening, which is an essential part of good communication, and how to recognize non-verbal communication, as in body language.

Practice Active Listening

In the last chapter, you learned a lot about how to communicate what you are feeling and how your chronic pain is impacting your life. As you already know, this is so important because it allows your healthcare providers to give you the best possible care. You can employ all that you learned there with your inner circle as well.

Use your words! Remember to be clear. Be honest. Let people know what you need, and give them the opportunity to help you. And once you have done all of that, listen! Your ability to actively listen to what others, especially your loved ones, are communicating back to you, will strengthen your relationships in so many ways.

While it may feel like they don't care or they aren't hearing you, maybe what they are trying to say is, "I'm doing my best." When you allow yourself to hear others and truly understand what they are saying, it gives you a base to build from and move forward in a way that works for everyone.

Here are a few tips to help you become a more active listener:

Listen to hear, not to respond

You've probably heard this before, and you've probably felt yourself doing it. It is common for most people to listen to respond. Don't beat yourself up for doing this; your intentions are good. Simply recognize when you are doing it. Take a moment.

Listen to their words

How are they speaking to you? Are their words strong or more passive? Are they repeating certain parts? They may be doing this because they are feeling unheard and don't know how to effectively communicate with you. Listen to what they are saying, and if you don't feel like you understand what they mean, ask them to rephrase it.

Listen to their tone of voice

A simple sentence like "I am hurt" can be said in so many different ways. It can be said quietly. It can be said forcefully. It can be yelled. It can be hard to get out. How does the tone communicate more about the situation to you? If that last statement is aggressive, it could also mean that whatever had hurt them has also made them incredibly angry, which could be clouding their judgement and signalling for a break in the conversation.

Observe their body language

We live in the words from morning till night, but there is so much more to communication if you are open to seeing it. Body language tells a story too; for example, posture, eye focus, and hand gestures. These all add extra information to the words that are being spoken, both by you and by them.

Let them know they have been heard

Sometimes all that is needed is just to listen and to acknowledge that you have heard what has been said. There are two ways that you can do this:

1. Listen and reflect – Repeat the content and share your understanding of the emotion behind what was said. Responding to content and emotion can help communication move forward, and break down walls, allowing for more expression of feelings and thoughts.

2. Seek more information – When you are not certain about what has been said or what is wanted of you, it's important to ask for clarification. It will help you listen more effectively and respond when you need to.

Minimize Conflict

"Practice the pause. Pause before judging. Pause before assuming. Pause before accusing. Pause whenever you're about to react harshly, and you'll avoid doing and saying things you'll later regret."
– Lori Deschene

Communication is a two-way street. Your responsibility in this is to make certain that the lines of communication are open. One of the best ways to maintain healthy communication with the ones you love, your friends, and your colleagues is to minimize conflict. I'm not saying that you have to ignore situations that make you angry or sad; what I am saying is that you can always find a way to communicate more effectively when you understand why you are feeling the way you are feeling.

Here are a few tools to help you be clearer in your communication:

Shift the focus

When things get heated, you can lose sight of what the original discussion was meant to be about. When that happens, it's time to bring the conversation back to the original topic. You may say something like: "I feel like we have drifted from the original point of this discussion." You might also suggest setting up another time to discuss the other things that are coming up, but ask that you stay on topic in this moment.

Buy time

When you find yourself getting very upset, you should stop yourself from reacting in the moment. Take time to calm down and think things through, so that you can approach the situation from a place of understanding. Give yourself the opportunity to reply thoughtfully rather than in the heat of the moment.

Understand the other's point of view

A good way to do this is to summarize what you have heard and ask for clarification. Really attempt to place yourself in the shoes of the person you are speaking to. Try to think through their ideas and truly understand them. This certainly helps develop tolerance and empathy for others.

Look for compromise

In many cases, there isn't a perfect solution or the ability to achieve total agreement; however, finding middle ground is always a possibility. Let go of what you don't really need.

Say you are sorry

Have you ever felt like you've hurt someone you love, and it was completely unintentional on your part? This happens so often. You might wish you could take back what you have either said or done, but you know you can't. Still, you might struggle to apologize because you didn't mean to cause the pain, and so, therefore, you don't feel like it's really your fault. Or it makes you feel weak. Or it bruises your ego.

So many relationships suffer for prolonged periods of time because we are unable to say we are sorry. This is an essential social skill. Saying you are sorry is not a sign of weakness; instead, it's a sign of courage and generosity. Apologizing brings healing to both yourself and the other person. Being sorry and forgiving are two very healing tools for the spirit.

Get the Support You Need

Your inner circle of family, friends, and colleagues want to help, but sometimes they don't always know how to help, and other times they may even help in ways that make things worse. Do not assume that others know what you want because "they should know." Tell them what you need them to know. In the last chapter, you began building a deeper understanding of your pain to be able to communicate it to your healthcare providers. You can combine that knowledge with the listening skills we just talked about, to become the best communicator you can be. You cannot change the communication of others; however, you can change your style of communication to be sure you are as clear as you can be.

- Be clear.
- Be honest.
- Be upfront!

Ask for Support

Giving and receiving help is a part of being in supportive relationships. Not being able to receive assistance can create unnecessary problems. We all need help sometimes, and I understand it is sometimes difficult to ask for it.

It may be difficult to admit that we are unable to do things for ourselves, or to be a burden to someone else. Part of being able to have strong relationships is being able to give and receive within our capacity. The ability to receive also gives the gift of the other party being able to freely give.

Ask for the support you need. The other person always has the right to decline giving you the support because it isn't within their capacity. This is okay. This is healthy. Create an open dialogue that allows for a truthful exchange. If the person you've asked for help can't give you what you need, ask them what they can do, and seek out others who can help you with the rest.

The first step to receiving support is admitting it. You are not a burden. Your loved ones want to help you. Give them that gift by being clear about what you need.

Decline Support

Your support circle may be incredibly helpful. However, if this leaves you feeling like you are dependent or incapable of doing things for yourself, and is directly affecting your self-esteem, then you can say *no* to the help offered. A simply worded message declining support can help without embarrassing the other person. This may sound like:

"Thank you for being so considerate, but today I think I can handle this myself. I hope I can take you up on the offer another time."

It's important to acknowledge the importance of the request. In this way, the person can see that you are declining the request, not the person.

Accept Support

Be prepared to accept support by having a specific answer, by knowing what you need support with. Rather than saying, "I don't know," or, "Thank you, but I don't need any help," you can say:

"Thank you; I don't need help making dinner, but I do need help buying the heavy groceries because I have trouble getting them into and out of the car."

Or,

"Thank you for the offer to bring over dinner, but maybe we could make dinner together. I could use the company and a friend to talk to."

Often, I have heard my clients say that their close family and friends should know what they need and that they shouldn't have to tell them. This makes for the beginning of many misunderstandings. Even the people who love you the most cannot read your mind, so you do have to tell them what you need.

When you give those around you a task that they can easily accomplish and which makes your life easier, you are really giving them a gift. People love being helpful and to know they have made a positive difference to someone they care about.

Communication Is Key

Communication is key to getting the support you need. That is the bottom line. Without the ability to clearly describe your pain, talk about your needs, ask for help, and listen to what others are saying to you, you will not be able to effectively advocate for yourself.

I understand that sometimes this is hard. It's not only your pain getting in the way but all of the emotions that pain causes. But keep on working at it. If you feel you are not being heard, take some time to figure out why. Often, there could be a break in the communication.

When you become an excellent communicator and active listener, you become a powerful self-manager for your chronic pain.

Chapter 10

An Integrated Approach to Chronic Pain

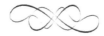

"Chronic pain is not all about the body, and it's not all about the brain — it's everything. Target everything. Take back your life."
– Sean Mackey MD PhD

This book reflects a deep personal journey. I offer my insights on life and dealing with chronic pain personally and professionally, and approach chronic pain from the perspective of a wellness coach, yogini, and physiotherapist, noting that your chronic pain has physical, mental, and emotional dimensions that need to be addressed. Your well-being entails a holistic approach, and you need many healthcare professionals to administer your health needs with an umbrella of care. How you navigate this is dependent on you becoming your own strong and informed self-advocate and the most effective self-manager.

Here is a summary of key points to keep in mind as you navigate your course in healing your chronic pain:

Tools for YOU

Discipline

Life is difficult, but sometimes we make life more difficult. Having discipline is not about accomplishing a series of "have to's." Sometimes our attachment to the word "discipline" drives us to constantly do something or feel guilty about not doing it. Although life is difficult, we do not have to approach it by being difficult ourselves. Defining it as a harsh reality or a pleasant reality does not prove helpful; it is just as it is. Adopting practices that ground you and leave you feeling empowered is key. Your practice then is discipline in action. This is different from task-oriented behaviour. Bringing your full attention to your practice, is falling into an experience of getting to know yourself. Apply yourself authentically and make all life your practice. Practice is not about what you get; it is about what you give. Whether you are driven or resistant, the medicine is the same: Do what is truly possible with unwavering commitment to giving yourself to the moment. Without this intention, practice becomes another task to be completed, and loses its ability to transform. And transformation, or freedom, is the reason for all discipline.

Practice Suggestions

- Do one thing at a time.
- Commit yourself to doing what is possible. Make a list of what you have to do tomorrow, eliminate activities that are unnecessary, and reschedule those that can and should be postponed.
- Take a nap when you need it.
- Slow down. Begin each activity with one gentle inhalation, followed by a calm exhalation.
- Ask for help with the task.
- When you notice that you are pushing yourself to complete a task, be kind with yourself. Inhale quietly and exhale gently, extending the very same kindness to yourself that you would extend to another in the same situation. Begin again.

Non-Judgement

- Are you aware of your internal dialogue?
- Is it negative or positive?
- Is it creating an inner conflict or inspiring you to do better for yourself?
- How are you interacting with yourself with your family and with your friends?

Begin to pay attention to how often you judge yourself. When I took this on as a personal practice, I was appalled to learn that most of the time my inner dialogue was self-judgmental. But what really shocked me was when I discovered something even more disconcerting: There was no way that I could be harsh toward myself and at the same time be compassionate to others. I realized also that the process of silently putting myself down was actually a form of egoism. If you expect more from yourself than from others, you're saying that you are better than others and therefore must perform at a superior level. I don't mean that you shouldn't set goals for yourself.

Rather, the question is, how do you react if you cannot meet these goals? Honestly admitting that you may not have done your best, is not judgment. It is judgement when you draw a conclusion about yourself based on your ideas about failure. Honesty involves taking responsibility; judgement has to do with blame. To view yourself as bad or a failure because you did not accomplish what you set out to do, is judgment. To state clearly and simply that you did not accomplish your plan, is taking responsibility.

It is important to bring a sense of comfort to your inner life, to your thoughts. Be aware of how you frame your reality and how you speak to yourself. When you resort to self-judgment, you are no longer present; you're no longer practicing. Learning to be present to yourself and to abide in that which is steady and comfortable, does not allow space for self-judgment. When you live this way, you are living fully.

A Self-Practice

If you are to free yourself self of thoughts of self-judgment, first you must be aware of them. Try this exercise. Taking your physical limitations and health into account, pick an activity that is difficult but not impossible for you to do. Practice, or rather attempt to practice, this every day for a short period of time. To begin, say silently or aloud, "I am attempting something difficult, and I appreciate myself for trying."

169

Then pay close attention to your internal dialogue as you go through your practice. At times, you may even talk yourself through your practice. Listen to the instructions you give yourself about the physical aspects of what you're doing. Whose instructions are those? Your own? A teacher's?

What do you say to yourself when you succeed? When you fail? When you are somewhere in between? Can you do your practice just to do the practice? Can your dialogue become agreeable? Is your practice quiet and steady? When you come out of your practice, say aloud:

"I have tried something difficult, and I appreciate myself for trying."

When you feel comfortable with your practice, pick another and repeat the process. Then try something that is difficult in another area of your life. Remember, the difficulty might never change, but your attitude and inner dialogue can.

Other practice suggestions:

- You can write down your internal dialogue right after your practice. Keep your notes brief. Do not try to interpret them. It will be interesting to note how the dialogue changes over time.
- If you are forcing a practice, ask yourself if this is in the true spirit of what you would like to achieve. If you notice that someone else is judging you, don't be quick to agree or to internalize the judgment. Think about what happened and agree only if this assessment aligns with yours.
- If you're going into a situation that makes you feel anxious, tense, or afraid, say to yourself, "I am perfect just as I am."

Intentions to abide by:

- I commit to just being myself.
- Perfection is an illusion.
- I am attempting something difficult, and I appreciate myself for trying.
- I am perfect just as I am.
- I am choosing to let go of my self-judgement now.

Faith

As I mentioned the word faith, this might create a sense of unease in some, as some may think that in order to have faith, one needs to be religious. Faith does not have to be just that; it's a belief in something bigger than yourself. Faith creates such a quality in your consciousness. It makes you solid and stable. Fear creates doubt, making you fearful, uncertain, and vulnerable. Faith integrates and consolidates your energy, whereas doubt scatters and disseminates your energy. To cultivate faith, one needs to integrate a certain set of behaviours, and one of them is discipline. Out of a faithful, disciplined behaviour, an equanimity can arise.

In order to commit ourselves to living integrated, full lives, we must have faith that our intentions are fruitful, and are meant to show us our central wholeness. Faith is a recipe made up of part trusting ourselves, part experience of life working out, and part intuitive connection with the divine. Knowing this about faith, instills assurance in the faithful. Faith has an innocence and a certainty to it.

Faith is said to be the quiet cousin of courage. Faith is willing to put its foot out when there is no guarantee that there will be a step to support it. Without faith, we cannot make the most important decisions in life.

What are we to have faith in? Basically, we ought to have faith in just about everything. The mystery of the universe and our existence in it demands faith in everything from the mundane to the spectacular.

The book *A Zen Harvest* includes this Japanese folk saying, which reminds us of the necessity of faith:

> Everything
> Changes in this world
> May flowers will open
> Each spring
> Just as usual.

Unless we have faith in the ability of these methods to facilitate self-transformation, we will be unable to continue them when the going gets difficult, boring, or demanding. Having faith in yourself honours that inner knowing that guides you unerringly home to the Divine.

Letting Go

Letting it go is difficult for most of us to understand and to practice. It does not mean not being involved or being uninterested; actually, these are opposites. If you are uninterested, you are drawn back or turned back on life, which in no way denies the difficulty of life. To let go is to be able to stand in the middle of the marketplace, with all its confusion and noise, and to remain present to yourself to all that is. Suffering usually comes from our attachment to things around us, so if you ask yourself what exactly you are to be detached from, the only possible answer is that you are to give up your attachment to the way you think things are. When you do, you get out of your own way and can experience another perspective.

Perspective

We can benefit from maintaining perspective about what is happening in life, at the present moment, right here, right now. When we cling to one point of view, we limit our ability to see what is in front of us. Life will continue to challenge us, and if we pay attention, we can allow these challenges to broaden our perspectives. Discrimination helps us make healthy choices in life. Stepping back and quietly contemplating what we really want in life can initiate actions in that direction. The choices we make now, determine our future.

In any action, it is important to know who or where we are now (our current state), where we want to go (direction), and the steps necessary to get there. How we react to touchy situations can provide valuable information about our deep behavioural patterns. Recognizing the existence of our discomfort or pain, identifying its cause, and then working to consciously weaken that cause, will eventually eliminate suffering.

Creating a new story for yourself is a chance to give yourself a new perspective. Here are some examples of stories that have helped me recently:

- I look for the light in each person.
- I need only simple, nourishing foods.
- Be with any fear or emotion.
- I am deeply committed to the results I want to create.
- Movement and the outdoors light me up.
- I care for my life by tending to finances, my health, and messages to people I care about.
- I enjoy sitting in stillness and quiet.

What stories would cause a powerful perspective shift for you?

Courage

"The opposite of courage isn't cowardice. It's conformity."
– Anonymous

I think, after the ability to love oneself and others, courage is the second most important quality to cultivate in life. We are constantly faced with the importance of true courage, which can be seen as equal parts: knowing what is possible for you and understanding your interdependence with the world around you. The times when I have been the most afraid, I felt disconnected from God, from spirit, from the universe, from family and friends, and most importantly, from my own heart—courage cannot exist in isolation. Contemplate and understand that when you do what is possible, you are not in free fall but are cradled by your bonds with the world around you. Your work is to distinguish what is important enough to require your commitment and what is not worthy of your courage. You can rest assured that when you act from true courage, the people, the tools, and your own inner knowing—all that is needed for the heroine's journey—will be available to you.

- Intentions for daily living:
- I will do what is possible.
- My courage is an expression of my love.
- Courage is the willingness to act in the face of the unknown.
- Being fully in each moment is a radical form of courage.
- Letting go of what I cannot change celebrates my courage.

Relaxation

You may have heard and read about relaxation as a pain management technique, but you may still be confused as to what relaxation is, its benefits, and how to achieve it. Relaxation involves using techniques to reduce or eliminate tension from both the body and the mind. Relaxation usually involves improved quality of sleep, better breathing, and less stress, anxiety, and pain. It often also instills a feeling of calm and well-being.

One of the most shocking effects I encountered when trying to employ relaxation techniques, was how unrelenting my thoughts were. I learned to relax my body, but my mind was still charging around from past to present to future and back again, in a turbulent flow of ideas and judgments. I realized that what was happening was not a mistake but a gift. By letting go of my physical tension, I could experience my mental tension. As I continued to practice breathwork with meditation, I was able to calm my mind and become less aware of my thoughts, and I was less controlled by them. Gradually, this awareness began to stay with me. Don't believe your thoughts; they are just neurotransmitters linking into receptor sites. They are not reality.

As I practiced, I got to see that this emerging freedom from the tyranny of my thoughts was the only real freedom. The key, even if the thoughts are there, is to not identify with them. By watching thoughts of anger, greed, boredom, and impatience, I was no longer at the mercy of them. I had some space to choose what I would say and do, in a way I never had before, and I began to recognize patterns. I began to take it all more lightly. By learning to relax, I experienced less physical tension, which allowed me to see my monkey mind, which allowed me to let go of it a bit, which allowed me to feel more connected to the present moment, which is another word for the infinite. Starting from the simple act of lying down to relax, I found a critical tool for living more in the present, with less tension and fear, and with more compassion for myself and others.

Intentions for daily living:

- Never pass up a chance to do nothing.
- I will nourish myself by making time for a 20-minute relaxation every day.
- If I think that I don't have time today for a 20-minute relaxation, that is a sure sign that I really need it.
- Relaxation is different from sleep, and I need both every day.
- A basic relaxation pose is an act of love and courage.

Chronic Pain and Your Relationships

Compassion

We can strengthen our ability to be compassionate by repeatedly expressing compassion. But compassion does not develop in isolation from the rest of our lives. What is compassion? Who should receive our compassion? When? How do we learn to hear the cries of the world? In the yoga sutras by Patanjali, he implies that compassion is to be expressed to everyone all the time. He promises that to do so will purify us. Expressing compassion is definitely a learn-as-you-go process. It is also cumulative. The old axiom that charity begins at home is so true—with compassion, you must begin with yourself. To be compassionate toward others, you must first understand that you suffer. This awareness allows you to see that others suffer too, and to respond with clarity to this condition, which is shared by all living beings.

One of the world's most well-known spiritual teachers came from India. He was called Buddha, or the awakened one. In his first teaching after his enlightenment, he imported the four noble truths. The basis of all Buddhist teaching goes straight to the heart of the matter of being alive to the truth of suffering, the truth of the origin of suffering, and the truth of the path that leads to the end of suffering. When we act from a heart of compassion, we always know what to do.

Intentions for daily living:

- I have compassion for myself. I have compassion for others.
- When I act from a heart of compassion, I always know what to do.
- Compassion comes from clarity and creates clarity.
- If you plant compassion, you get compassion.

Control

When we attempt to control things around us, although it engages us with life, it really affects and blocks us from connecting with others and with ourselves.

Consider this: The more we try to control our world, the less control we have .The more we are willing to let go of control and simply stay present with what is, the more control we have.

Intentions for daily living:

- The only real control I have is the choice of my own thoughts, my own words, and my own actions.
- I choose how I react. I do not have to react right now.
- Control is the greatest illusion.

What can I let go of right now?

Fear

In my experience, I feel we live with two basic emotions: fear and love. However, there are many aspects to each. Take greed for an example. Greed springs from the fear that there isn't enough for whatever you need. Another aspect of fear is anger, which is actually an attempt to defend against the harm that you perceive is coming. One of the most interesting things about fear is that it exists in relationship to the future. Is it possible to live without fear? I doubt it, and it may not even be desirable. Fear is useful; it warns us of potential danger and acts as a self-preservation device in this post-modern era. But most fears are not about being attacked by wild animal in the woods; instead, we fear illness, loneliness, and poverty. These and other fears can either run our lives or be viewed as part of our human condition. We can choose to observe our feelings on a daily basis, and continually bring awareness back to what is happening in the present moment so that we can look more completely.

Patience

Have patience with the process. Often, there is little we can control. Allowing ourselves to go with the flow of life rather than paddling upstream instills a feeling of calm and patience and contentment. Impatience feeds anxiety and can snowball into a host of negative feelings and thoughts. Becoming aware of this takes practice and the act of letting go.

Intentions for daily living:

- Is the problem the situation or my reaction to the situation?
- Everything is moving at the proper speed.
- Choice is the most profound freedom.

- There is always enough time in nature.
- It won't always be like this.

Non-Attachment

"The secret of happiness lies in the minds
released from worldly ties."
– Buddha

When we develop an attachment to things, we can lose perspective and start to use these external things to define us. It's important to realize that the ups and downs of life come and go, people come and go, and so do situations. Having attachments often grows into cravings, and not experiencing a certain kind of situation or object will upset us. Having an attitude of unattachment of non-entanglement to things creates a situation where your happiness is not defined by the presence or absence of it.

Intentions for daily living:

- Will this be important in a year? In five years?
- Things are as they are.
- What will happen if I don't get what I want right now?
- This is just a thought.
- How should it be?

Suffering

There is a difference between pain and suffering. Physical, emotional, and mental pain are inevitable in life. Suffering is another matter. Suffering is the personalization we bring to our difficulties. For example, we blame others for our pain, or we feel sorry for ourselves because of the pain.

Intentions for daily living:

- Who is suffering?
- Release all suffering, and love life right now.
- It may be difficult, but I do not need to suffer.
- That's part of it too.

Service and Our Connection to the Whole

Connection

I hope you agree that the most powerful human drive is the one for connection. Even though we may not always know how to express our yearning for connection, nonetheless, we long for it—with other humans and with that mystery we call God or the universe. We long for this connection because we feel incomplete without the meaning it provides in our lives. This driving need shapes our lives, in ways both large and small. We may at times feel disconnected, but we can rest in the certainty that all beings and all things are interconnected.

Your perception and how you relate to the world is dependent on your experiences. You, like all humans, have experiences that separate you from life. This experience has formed your beliefs about the world and yourself, and your reactions to them. Whatever filters through, you call reality. But is it? Your reality is subjective. The most important thing about perception is that it can change, and it is relative to individuals, to time, to places, and to contexts. We can perceive ourselves as separate beings or as being profoundly interconnected with everything around us. The more we experience ourselves as being separate, the more we long for connection.

We may seek connection in ways that are not productive, such as drugs, alcohol, promiscuous sex, or damaging relationships. And other times, we may run from connection by being busy, but none of these strategies help us discover the interconnectedness of all of life. Each of us has a purpose, something to contribute to life. Perhaps happiness is the state that we feel when we find what it is that we can contribute with joy to the world. When we embrace our importance, we are living our connection with others and the world around us. In this state, we can change the world. Just a kind gesture or a generous word can change another state. Stopping to pay attention to what another person means, and helping when appropriate, can change that person's life. Connection is that process of knowing our importance to all, as well as comprehending that others share this importance with us.

Breathing and Chronic Pain

An expression in India states that there are more than 40 different ways to breathe, whereas most Westerners think there are only two (inhale and exhale). Vedic scientists have studied and worked with breathing as a healing modality for thousands of years, combining mental imagery with abdominal breathwork. Although few, if any, studies have investigated the relationship between abdominal breathing and the treatment of chronic pain, energy healers who treat patients with a host of diseases use breathwork as the core of their energy work.

(Rosen, 2002; Swayzee, 1998). Rosen describes a concept called Bandha, a series of respiratory contractions to unlock the cause of pain. It is also suggested by healers that clients not merely practice abdominal breathing but combine imagery with breathwork, and visualize inhaling and exhaling through that area for pain relief.

Benefits Of Breathing/Pranayama

1. Decreases resting heart rate
2. Promotes feelings of relaxation
3. Decreases muscle tension
4. Improves mental clarity
5. Increases oxygen capacity in lungs
6. Helps deal with stress overload

Meditation and Chronic Pain

"Empty the cup."
– Zen Master Nan-in

Your mind is a thought generating organ. Thought forms perpetually arise in your awareness. If you try to stop your thoughts with the intention of creating stillness in your mind, your mental activity may quiet for a few moments, but it will almost certainly start up again at full speed. The activity in your mind is communicated to every cell in your body. When your mind is turbulent, your messenger molecules communicate turbulence to your cells, tissues, and organs. If you can quiet your mind, you can send messages of peace and harmony to every cell in your body. Meditation is the technology that enables you temporary elite escape from the cycle. Through the process of gently focusing your attention while innocently witnessing the thought forms that come and go in your mind, you enter into the gap between thoughts, cleansing the domain of unbound awareness, and taking your mind from constricted to expanded awareness.

Many people recognize the name of Jon Kabat-Zinn as the country's greatest proponent of mindfulness meditation, but many do not know that his career in this field began by focusing on the response to pain relief through meditation. Through this work, Kabat-Zinn found substantial evidence for nonmedical pain relief through the Zen practice of mindfulness meditation. Since then, others have replicated his findings, most recently Marone and colleagues. Although pain may seem like a physical phenomenon, the mind-body-spirit paradigm suggests that by involving the mind in spirit, with pain relief, the cause of the problem as well as the symptoms may be lessened, if not eradicated all together. Whereas Kabat-Zinn's method of mindfulness utilizes association, getting in touch and comfortable with the pain, others advocate the use of meditation exclusively to disassociate from pain as a means of temporary relief.

Yoga and Chronic Pain

Back pain is one of the most common maladies to affect people older than the age of 25. Prolonged sitting and standing posture, weak stomach muscles, and athletic activities top the list of factors contributing to chronic low back pain. Many people find little or no relief from standard medical practices and are turning to yoga as an alternative or complementary modality, particularly in regard to sacroiliac joint problems and lower back pain. By stretching tight muscles and balancing the strength and flexibility of the muscle supporting the joints where pain originates, yoga can be a positive and inexpensive means to reduce and eliminate joint pain. Yoga has been found to be helpful for a variety of health-related problems, including carpal tunnel syndrome.

Music Therapy and Chronic Pain

Just as several theories attempt to explain the nature of music's relaxing qualities, so do various theories purport to explain music's ability to reduce pain.

The most obvious one suggests that music acts as a diversion, by distracting one's thoughts from the original pain. The dissociation from pain offers temporary relief. In regard to healing vibrations, the entrainment theory is called upon once again to explain music's ability to decrease pain, with healing sounds providing a stronger vibration than the energy created by neural pain. Music's healing quality likely combines these two aspects. Current research into approaches utilizing sound vibration, entrainment, and cancer, continues to show promise in the search for a cancer cure and other immune system illnesses.

In his book, *The Healing Power of Sound*, Dr. Mitchell Gaynor discusses the use of music in a variety of healing parameters. Gaynor cites several studies, including research that shows the relationship between music and pain-relieving opiates. Even though music as medicine is not considered mainstream therapy yet, Deena Spear (2002) thinks it's only a matter of time. As a violin maker and acoustic researcher, Spear has been involved with many healing sessions and has observed many amazing results of pain reduction through music.

When we think of pain, we need to go beyond just the physical manifestations of pain, for there are mental and emotional manifestations as well. I truly believe that we are all in some degree of physical, mental. and emotional pain. How much this impacts our daily lives and function probably determines whether you will address it or not. If you are reading or listening to this book at this point, then I take it you are looking for answers and transformation.

Realize that there are common threads to human suffering, and they manifest in anxiety, depression, sleep issues, nutritional issues, and many more, which have been conditions that have been experienced by the human race for eons. Of course, the world has changed, bringing in different environmental stressors, but there are solutions that have been discovered too, and you are not alone in your journey.

Commit to taking your power back in all areas that you can control. This book provides a good foundation to begin, and I hope that this is the beginning of deep self-healing and, through your experience, you will empower others to do the same.

My own journey has been a deeply spiritual one and, as I delve deeper, I realize I am just at the very beginning and there are mysteries and mysticism to tap into that opens up dimensions that I didn't know existed. Begin with self-exploration and commit to understanding your role in this. By comprehending that human beings are energy, one can begin to comprehend new ways of viewing health and illness.

About the Author

Theven Sabga has over 30 years of experience as a physiotherapist, helping countless clients manage their chronic pain. During those years, she realized that pain management is much more than just managing the physical symptoms. Her clients' frustration became hers as she worked to understand why they weren't getting the care they needed. This led her to develop an effective three-month coaching program where she uses her four-step framework to guide her clients in becoming effective self-managers and self-advocates. Ultimately, *Heal Your Chronic Pain* empowers you by placing you back in the driver's seat so you can live a healthy and fulfilling life.

While she was growing up in South Africa, Theven's father ignited a spirituality in her that continues to guide her in all that she does today. After moving to Canada in her twenties, Theven experienced challenges that asked her to re-examine her sense of self, and how life has guided her to learn more about how to help those close to her, but also her clients, to achieve greater health through addressing all aspects of themselves: spiritual, emotional, and physical.

In her pursuit of constant growth, Theven has achieved her BSC Pt and worked in Capetown South Africa, and completed her postsecondary education in manual therapy and acupuncture in Toronto. Theven is a yoga teacher, meditation teacher, and a Master Wellness Coach with the International Coaches of Wellness Professionals, where she continues to also train coaches in the practice.

All of this knowledge and experience has led her to this point where she can now help her clients achieve a deep approach to healing in all aspects of their life, ultimately helping them successfully manage their chronic pain.

Theven shares this work not only in her program, but in her writing. She is currently working on her second book. Her goal is to share all that she has learned with as many people as possible, so that they too can live happier, healthier and more fulfilling lives.

If you are ready to take control of your chronic pain and step into a happier, healthier and more fulfilling life, there are many ways you can work with Theven. There is her three-month program, Heal Your Chronic Pain, which will provide you with a unique roadmap for your healing journey. She also offers online yoga classes, as well as virtual and in-person wellness coaching sessions, and individual or group meditation classes both virtual or in person.

Follow Theven on social media for upcoming workshops. (facebook : Well Awareness, Instagram: well.awareness, websites: healyourchronicpain.com and www.wellawareness.ca)

Made in the USA
Monee, IL
11 December 2022